# Management of Melanoma of the Head and Neck

*Editor*

AL HAITHAM AL SHETAWI

## ORAL AND MAXILLOFACIAL SURGERY CLINICS OF NORTH AMERICA

www.oralmaxsurgery.theclinics.com

*Consulting Editor*
RUI P. FERNANDES

May 2022 • Volume 34 • Number 2

**ELSEVIER**

1600 John F. Kennedy Boulevard • Suite 1800 • Philadelphia, Pennsylvania, 19103-2899

http://www.oralmaxsurgery.theclinics.com

**ORAL AND MAXILLOFACIAL SURGERY CLINICS OF NORTH AMERICA Volume 34, Number 2**
**May 2022 ISSN 1042-3699, ISBN-13: 978-0-323-84995-1**

Editor: John Vassallo; j.vassallo@elsevier.com
Developmental Editor: Jessica Nicole B. Cañaberal

*Oral and Maxillofacial Surgery Clinics of North America* (ISSN 1042-3699) is published quarterly by Elsevier Inc., 360 Park Avenue South, New York, NY 10010-1710. Months of issue are February, May, August, and November. Business and Editorial Offices: 1600 John F. Kennedy Blvd., Suite 1800, Philadelphia, PA 19103-2899. Periodicals postage paid at New York, NY and additional mailing offices. Subscription prices are $405.00 per year for US individuals, $961.00 per year for US institutions, $100.00 per year for US students/residents, $478.00 per year for Canadian individuals, $990.00 per year for Canadian institutions, $100.00 per year for Canadian students/residents, $530.00 per year for international individuals, $990.00 per year for international institutions and $235.00 per year for international students/residents. To receive student/resident rate, orders must be accompanied by name or affiliated institution, date of term, and the *signature* of program/residency coordinator on institution letterhead. Orders will be billed at individual rate until proof of status is received. Foreign air speed delivery is included in all *Clinics* subscription prices. All prices are subject to change without notice. **POSTMASTER:** Send address changes to *Oral and Maxillofacial Surgery Clinics of North America,* Elsevier Periodicals **Customer Service, 11830 Westline Industrial Drive, St. Louis, MO 63146. Tel: 1-800-654-2452 (U.S. and Canada); 314-447-8871 (outside U.S. and Canada). Fax: 314-447-8029. E-mail: journalscustomerservice-usa@elsevier.com (for print support); journalsonlinesupport-usa@elsevier.com (for online support)**.

*Reprints.* For copies of 100 or more, of articles in this publication, please contact the Commercial Reprints Department, Elsevier Inc., 360 Park Avenue South, New York, NY 10010-1710. Tel.: 212-633-3874; Fax: 212-633-3820; Email: reprints@elsevier.com.

*Oral and Maxillofacial Surgery Clinics of North America* is covered in *MEDLINE/PubMed* (*Index Medicus*), *Science Citation Index Expanded (SciSearch®)*, *Journal Citation Reports/Science Edition*, and *Current Contents®/Clinical Medicine*.

# Contributors

## CONSULTING EDITOR

**RUI P. FERNANDES, MD, DMD, FACS, FRCS(Ed)**
Clinical Professor and Chief, Division of Head and Neck Surgery, Program Director, Head and Neck Oncologic Surgery and Microvascular Reconstruction Fellowship, Departments of Oral and Maxillofacial Surgery, Neurosurgery, and Orthopaedic Surgery and Rehabilitation, University of Florida Health Science Center, University of Florida College of Medicine, Jacksonville, Florida, USA

## EDITOR

**AL HAITHAM AL SHETAWI, MD, DMD, FACS**
Division of Surgical Oncology, Department of Surgery, Chief, Division of Oral and Maxillofacial Surgery, Vassar Brothers Medical Center, Nuvance Health, Dyson Center for Cancer Care, Poughkeepsie, New York, USA

## AUTHORS

**AL HAITHAM AL SHETAWI, MD, DMD, FACS**
Division of Surgical Oncology, Department of Surgery, Chief, Division of Oral and Maxillofacial Surgery, Vassar Brothers Medical Center, Nuvance Health, Dyson Center for Cancer Care, Poughkeepsie, New York, USA

**VINESH ANANDARAJAN, MD**
Department of Surgery, Vassar Brothers Medical Center, Nuvance Health, Poughkeepsie, New York, USA

**R. BRYAN BELL, MD, DDS, FACS, FRCS(Ed)**
Physician Executive and Director, Division of Surgical Oncology, Radiation Oncology and Clinical Programs, Providence Cancer Institute of Oregon, Director of Surgical Oncology Research, Earle A. Chiles Research Institute, Portland, Oregon, USA

**VINCENT P. BELTRANI, MD**
Caremount Medical, Poughkeepsie, New York, USA

**ANTHONY M. BUNNELL, MD, DMD**
Division of Head and Neck Surgery, Department of Oral and Maxillofacial Surgery, University of Florida College of Medicine, Jacksonville, Florida, USA

**SRINIVASA RAMA CHANDRA, MD, BDS, FDSRCS (Eng), FIBCSOMS (Onc-Recon), FACS**
Associate Professor and Program Director, Oral and Maxillofacial Surgery, Oregon Health & Sciences University, Portland, Oregon, USA

**YASSER FARAJ, DO**
KCU-GME Consortium/ADCS Orlando Dermatology Program, Orlando, Florida, USA

**ZIPEI FENG, MD, PhD**
Department of Otolaryngology, Baylor College of Medicine, Department of Head and Neck Surgery, MD Anderson Cancer Center, Houston, Texas, USA

**RUI P. FERNANDES, MD, DMD, FACS, FRCS(Ed)**
Clinical Professor and Chief, Division of Head and Neck Surgery, Program Director, Head and Neck Oncologic Surgery and Microvascular Reconstruction Fellowship, Departments of Oral and Maxillofacial Surgery, Neurosurgery, and Orthopaedic Surgery and Rehabilitation, University of Florida Health Science Center, University of Florida College of Medicine, Jacksonville, Florida, USA

**JASON FOSTER, MD, FACS**
Professor of Surgery, Division of Surgical Oncology, University of Nebraska Medical Center, Omaha, Nebraska, USA

**MICA D.E. GLAUN, MD**
Department of Otolaryngology, Baylor College of Medicine, Department of Head and Neck Surgery, MD Anderson Cancer Center, Houston, Texas, USA

**KEVIN J. HARRINGTON, PhD**
Head and Neck Unit, The Royal Marsden Hospital, Division of Radiotherapy and Imaging, Targeted Therapy Team, The Institute of Cancer Research, London, United Kingdom

**EMILIE S. JACOBSEN, MD**
Divisions of Dermatologic Surgery and Dermatology, David Geffen School of Medicine, University of California, Los Angeles, Los Angeles, California, USA

**ARSHAD KALEEM, MD, DMD, FACS**
Assistant Professor, DeWitt Daughtry Family Department of Surgery, Division of Oral and Maxillofacial Surgery, Section of Head and Neck Surgical Oncology and Microvascular Reconstructive Surgery, University of Miami Miller School of Medicine, Jackson Health System, Miami, Florida, USA

**MIRIAM LANGO, MD**
Professor, Department of Head and Neck Surgery, MD Anderson Cancer Center, Houston, Texas, USA

**STACEY M. NEDRUD, MD, DMD**
Division of Head and Neck Surgery, Department of Oral and Maxillofacial Surgery, University of Florida College of Medicine, Jacksonville, Florida, USA

**PABLO NENCLARES, MD**
Head and Neck Unit, The Royal Marsden Hospital, Division of Radiotherapy and Imaging, Targeted Therapy Team, The Institute of Cancer Research, London, United Kingdom

**JAMES NITZKORSKI, MD, FSSO**
Department of Surgery, Vassar Brothers Medical Center, Nuvance Health, Dyson Center for Cancer Care, Poughkeepsie, New York, USA

**NEEL PATEL, MD, DMD**
Former Fellow, DeWitt Daughtry Family Department of Surgery, Division of Oral and Maxillofacial Surgery, Section of Head and Neck Surgical Oncology and Microvascular Reconstructive Surgery, University of Miami Miller School of Medicine, Jackson Health System, Miami, Florida, USA

**JAY PONTO, MD, DDS**
Fellow, Head and Neck Oncologic and Microvascular Reconstructive Surgery, Providence Cancer Institute, Portland, Oregon, USA

**SRAVANI SINGU, BS**
University of Nebraska Medical Center, College of Medicine, Omaha, Nebraska, USA

**TEO SOLEYMANI, MD, FAAD, FACMS**
Division of Dermatologic Surgery, Mohs Micrographic and Reconstructive Surgery, Dermatologic Oncology, Director, Pigmented Lesion and Melanoma Clinic, David Geffen School of Medicine, University of California, Los Angeles, Los Angeles, California, USA

**R.L. VIJAYARAGHAVAN, MD, DNB, FASNC**
Department of Molecular Imaging and Radionuclide Therapy, Nanjappa Life Care Super-Specialty Hospital, Shimoga, India

**KATHRYN WELLS, DO**
Department of Surgery, Vassar Brothers
Medical Center, Nuvance Health,
Poughkeepsie, New York, USA

**WILL WING, DO**
Department of Surgery, Dyson Center for
Cancer Care, Nuvance Health, Poughkeepsie,
New York, USA

# Contents

Melanoma is often initially evaluated by the dermatologist. A methodical evaluation requires complete history and detailed clinical physical examination and appropriate decisions regarding biopsies. Accurate diagnosis and staging require clinicopathologic correlation and an excellent relationship with the dermatopathologist. Subsequent definitive treatment may be managed entirely by the dermatologist or might require a multidisciplinary team of specialists.

The rates of melanoma continue to rise, with recent estimates have shown that 18% to 22% of new melanoma cases occur within the head and neck in the United States each year. The mainstay of treatment of nonmetastatic primary melanomas of the head and neck includes the surgical resection and management of regional disease as indicated. Thorough knowledge of the classification and staging of melanoma is paramount to evaluate prognosis, determine the appropriate surgical intervention, and assess eligibility for adjuvant therapy and clinic trials. The traditional clinicopathologic classification of melanoma is based on morphologic aspects of the growth phase and distinguishes 4 of the most common subtypes as defined by the World Health Organization: superficial spreading, nodular, acral lentiginous, and lentigo maligna melanoma. The data used to derive the AJCC TNM Categories are based on superficial spreading melanoma and nodular subtypes. Melanoma is diagnosed histopathologically following initial biopsy that will assist with classifying the tumor to guide treatment. Classification is based on tumor thickness and ulceration (T stage, Breslow Staging), Regional Lymph Node Involvement (N Stage), and presence of metastasis (M Stage). Tumor thickness (Breslow thickness) and ulceration are 2 independent prognostic factors that have been shown to be the strongest predictors of survival and outcome. Clark level of invasion and mitotic rate are no longer incorporated into the current AJCC staging system, but still have shown to be important prognostic factors for cutaneous melanoma. For patients with metastatic (Stage IV) disease Lactate Dehydrogenase remains an independent predictor of survival. The Maxillofacial surgeon must remain up to date on the most current management strategies in this patient population. Classification systems and staging provide the foundation for clinical decision making and prognostication for the Maxillofacial surgeon when caring for these patients.

Accurate diagnosis and staging of malignant melanoma remain crucial components in the overall treatment and prognosis of the patient. Advanced imaging modalities as well as laboratory testing continue to constitute an important part of the workup in melanoma and have seen several developments in recent years. The authors discuss imaging techniques and serum biomarkers used in the assessment of the melanoma patient.

Surgical management of head and neck melanoma starts from the primary biopsy of the cutaneous site by a narrow excision with a 1 to 3 mm margins. The margin should include the whole breadth and sufficient depth of the lesion. The key is not to transect the lesion. With the advent of molecular testing, gene expression profiling, and immunotherapies, the surgical management of advanced melanoma has changed. Sentinel lymph node biopsy is an essential armamentarium for T2a and higher staging/greater than 1 mm thick and advance stage disease. Molecular pathogenesis and cancer immunology are recognized in the recent treatment protocols along with surgery in advanced stages of melanoma.

Surgical excision achieving clear histologic margins remains the mainstay treatment for primary cutaneous melanoma. Tumors of the head and neck, particularly those arising in chronically sun-damaged skin, often demonstrate extensive and asymmetric subclinical extension. Over the decades, this has proven to be a significant problem for tumors arising on the head and neck, as anatomic and functional complexities of these areas have led to suboptimal surgical treatment, yielding unacceptably high rates of local recurrence and persistently positive margins with traditional wide local excision. Patients who undergo Mohs micrographic surgery may have improved survival over those who undergo wide local excision.

The utilization of sentinel lymph node (SLN) biopsy has transformed the workup and staging of intermediate-thickness cutaneous melanomas. SLN biopsy, performed at the time of primary tumor excision, accurately maps lymph nodes at risk of harboring occult metastatic deposits from head and neck cutaneous melanomas and represents the current standard of care. Completion lymphadenectomy identifies additional tumor in 12% to 24% of SLN biopsy positive cases but does not affect melanoma-specific survival.

The head and neck region is unique from the other anatomic sites due to its rich blood supply and ability to heal well after surgery. Surgical extirpation of melanoma usually requires wide resection margins, and the defect from surgery can be devastating to the patient and impossible to conceal sometimes. Therefore, the goal of a reconstructive technique is to restore the uniformity of skin color, texture, and contour and preserve the function. In general, head and neck skin defects are reconstructed with local and regional flaps. In this paper, the authors review the most common flaps used in head and neck reconstruction.

Head and neck mucosal melanomas are uncommon and aggressive malignancies that arise mainly in the nasal cavity and paranasal sinuses, with the next commonest site being the oral cavity. The mainstay of treatment is radical surgical resection.

Adjuvant radiotherapy improves locoregional control but does not improve overall survival. Systemic treatment with immunotherapy or targeted therapies can offer scope for modifying the course of the disease in both the adjuvant and the recurrent and metastatic setting. Further understanding of the genomic landscape and factors regulating immunogenicity will lead to further therapeutic opportunities in this challenging disease.

## Adjuvant and Neoadjuvant Therapies in Cutaneous Melanoma 315

Jay Ponto and R. Bryan Bell

Melanoma is the most common cause of skin cancer-related death in the United States. Cutaneous melanoma is most prevalent in the head and neck. The long-term prognosis has been poor and chemotherapy is not curative. Complete surgical resection with locally advanced disease can be challenging and melanoma is resistant to radiation. Advances made in immunotherapy and genomically targeted therapy have transformed the treatment of metastatic melanoma; as of 2021, the 5-year survival for metastatic melanoma is greater than 50%. Ongoing clinical studies are underway to integrate these life-saving therapies into the presurgical or postsurgical settings. This article reviews that effort.

## Future Treatments in Melanoma 325

Kathryn Wells, Vinesh Anandarajan, and James Nitzkorski

Melanoma is a highly malignant tumor that is relatively common in the United States. Surgical extirpation is the mainstay in treatment, but a multimodal therapeutic approach is increasingly important in the era of highly effective immune and targeted therapies. Although resection of melanoma will continue to be the mainstay of management for the conceivable future, improvements in multimodality therapy have and will continue to rewrite the therapeutic playbook for this lethal and increasingly complex malignancy for head and neck surgeons treating patients with melanoma.

# ORAL AND MAXILLOFACIAL SURGERY CLINICS OF NORTH AMERICA

# Preface

# Head and Neck Melanoma: Where Are We Now?

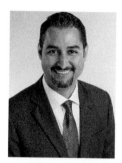

Al Haitham Al Shetawi, MD, DMD, FACS
*Editor*

This issue of the *Oral and Maxillofacial Surgery Clinics of North America* is devoted to the important topic of head and neck melanoma. There are some important facts about melanoma that make it a dedicated issue. The incidence of melanoma is rising faster than any other cancer. Melanoma accounts for only about 1% of skin cancers but causes the vast majority of skin cancer deaths. It is one of the most common forms of cancer in young people, especially among young women. There have been significant advancements in the field of melanoma over the past decade. These range from better understanding of immunology and immunopathology and improved diagnostic and surgical techniques to continued evolution of adjuvant therapies like immunotherapies and targeted therapies. In this issue, we review basic pathology, workup, staging, surgical and nodal management, reconstructive techniques, and adjuvant therapies. We have special topics on mucosal head and neck melanoma and future melanoma treatments. There is no doubt that the management of a melanoma patient is multidisciplinary

and incorporates many disciplines like dermatology, pathology, radiology, surgery, and medical oncology. I am thankful to all the outstanding experts in this issue from multiple disciplines who agreed to share their knowledge and expertise. It is impossible to cover all the advances in the field of melanoma, but in this issue of the *Oral and Maxillofacial Surgery Clinics of North America*, we attempted to provide the reader with an updated review on head and neck melanoma. I want to thank Dr Rui Fernandes for giving me the opportunity to assemble this issue.

Al Haitham Al Shetawi, MD, DMD, FACS
Division of Surgical Oncology, Division of Oral &
Maxillofacial Surgery, Departmet of Surgery,
Vassar Brothers Medical Center, Nuvance Health,
45 Reade Place, 3rd Floor, Dyson Center for
Cancer Care, Poughkeepsie, NY 12601, USA

*E-mail address:*
Al-haitham.al-shetawi@nuvancehealth.org

Oral Maxillofacial Surg Clin N Am 34 (2022) xi
https://doi.org/10.1016/j.coms.2021.11.009
1042-3699/22/© 2021 Published by Elsevier Inc.

# Preface

# Head and Neck Melanoma: Where Are We Now?

# Introduction to Head and Neck Melanoma
## A Dermatologist's Perspective

Yasser Faraj, DO[a],*, Vincent P. Beltrani, MD[b]

## KEYWORDS

- Melanoma • Pathogenesis • Risk factors • Melanoma of head and neck
- Superficial spreading melanoma • Nodular melanoma • Lentigo maligna melanoma

## KEY POINTS

- Thorough physical examination and history are of the utmost importance in the evaluation of skin lesions.
- All cell types of the dermis and subcutaneous tissue have the potential to proliferate into benign or malignant lesions.
- Not all pigmented lesions are melanocytic tumors, and not all melanocytic tumors are pigmented.

## INTRODUCTION

Many a patient's journey with melanoma begins at the dermatologist's office. Clinically suspicious lesions are either the "chief complaint" or discovered incidentally by the clinician performing a complete and thorough skin examination. It is critical to understand that patients with risk factors for skin cancer often have several skin cancers over a lifetime, and, although they are often intent on focusing on a specific lesion, it is incumbent upon the clinician to perform full skin examinations on a regular basis.

Dermatologists are faced with the task of evaluating numerous skin lesions on every patient. Although an experienced clinician can perform a detailed complete skin examination in mere minutes, the amount of information processed during this encounter is staggering. It is therefore critical to recognize how every facet of a thorough office visit is of great value in the evaluation of skin lesions.

### Chief Complaint

Dermatology is a unique and vast specialty in that pathology is evaluated from the top of the head to the soles of the feet, from the surface of the skin to the subcutaneous tissue and mucous membranes, in newborn infants and up to the elderly. The "chief complaint" for most patients presenting to a dermatologist is either an inflammatory process ("I have a rash") or a neoplastic process ("I have a growth"). Pathologic findings can be completely benign and indeed often cosmetic, or serious and potentially deadly.

### Medications/Allergies

Medications and allergies are always critical to patient's care. Not only does it give a glimpse at comorbidities but also it prepares us in the event that management requires additional medications. Concern over anticoagulants and skin surgery comes up frequently, but anticoagulation rarely needs to be interrupted for skin surgery.[1,2(p3)] In addition, perioperative antibiotics are rarely necessary unless true signs of infection exist.[3–8]

### History of Present Illness

The history of present illness is often the most critical part of the visit, and the following questions are routine regarding a given skin lesion:

[a] KCU-GME Consortium/ADCS Orlando Dermatology Program, Orlando, FL, USA; [b] Caremount Medical, Poughkeepsie, NY, USA
* Corresponding author. 15 West Colonial Drive, Unit 1314, Orlando, FL 32801.
E-mail address: yasserfaraj92@gmail.com

Oral Maxillofacial Surg Clin N Am 34 (2022) 213–220
https://doi.org/10.1016/j.coms.2021.11.007
1042-3699/22/© 2021 Elsevier Inc. All rights reserved.

- How long has it been present?
- changed in shape, size, color?
- Are there any symptoms (pain, bleeding, pruritus)?
- Have you ever had one like this before?
- any treatment to date?
- any previous history of skin cancer?
- lifetime sun exposure have you had?
- Do you typically burn or tan?[9–11]

It is critical to understand that an identical lesion on 2 different people may be considered quite differently. A 5-mm, evenly pigmented, well-demarcated macule would be clinically benign if it has been present since childhood in a 20-year-old patient with a dark complexion (Fitzpatrick skin type 4–5), while clinically worrisome if it is of recent onset and growing in size in a 60-year-old patient with red hair, blue eyes, freckles (Fitzpatrick skin type I-II), a history of skin cancer, a lifetime of excess sun exposure, and a family history of melanoma. For this reason, it is often difficult to render an accurate clinical diagnosis from a simple photograph.

### Review of System

The review of systems reflects a specific evaluation of relevant symptoms in other organ systems. For patients with clinically suspicious lesions, questions about weight loss, adenopathy, and other symptoms suggestive of metastatic disease are relevant.

### Past Medical History

Past medical history is relevant when considering comorbidities that impact management. Common examples include considering surgical procedures in poorly controlled diabetics or patients on anticoagulation therapy. Immunosuppressed patients are often at higher risk for skin cancer. In addition, patients with other serious comorbidities need to prioritize their treatments and consider less aggressive management if appropriate.

### Family History

Family history is also critically important, as an increased risk of skin cancer is often both genetic and generically associated with inherited skin type. Melanoma specifically has been linked to clinical syndromes[12–15] and genetic linkages.[16–18]

### Social History

Social history is relevant most importantly regarding questions about casual and occupational sun exposure. There is an increased risk of developing melanoma with an increasing number of sunburn episodes, and this correlation persists throughout the lifespan.[19–22] However, evidence suggesting the presence of "a critical age" at which sun exposure substantially increased risk of developing melanoma is inconsistent, and there seems to be no statistically significant correlation between the time of excessive sun exposure and the development of sun-induced melanoma.[22–24] In addition, exposure from tanning beds and other artificial UV radiation sources has also be shown to significantly increase the risk of developing melanoma and other skin cancers.[25–29] Smoking and alcohol abuse also result in negative skin changes like volume-related skin aging, inflammatory changes, and impaired wound healing.[30,31]

### Physical Examination

Physical examination (PE) is the most challenging and difficult part of a dermatologic visit. Excellent lighting and an examination table that allows for easy positioning of the patient are essential. One effective routine is to start on the right side of the patient while they are in a seated position and have them lean forward to examine their back. Then, the clinician can lay them in a partially reclined position with feet up to proceed with the right side of the body starting with the scalp and continuing down to the right foot before moving to examine the left foot and continuing up the left side of the body. It is interesting to note that the incidence of sun-induced tumors is greater on the left side of the face than the right side, presumably because of sun exposure while driving.[32,33]

During a dermatologic examination, the clinician will usually note numerous common skin lesions, and only with substantial experience will a clinician develop the necessary skill to easily identify most lesions. Although a detailed description of each lesion, an overview of describing each morphology, and a review of relevant dermatopathology is beyond the scope of this article, suffice it to say that any normal cell type found in the skin and subcutaneous tissue can proliferate into a benign or malignant skin tumor. These include keratinocytes, melanocytes, fibroblasts, sebocytes, eccrine and apocrine cells, follicular cells, myocytes, neural cells, and adipocytes (**Boxes 1 and 2**).

## IDENTIFICATION, EVALUATION, AND MANAGEMENT OF MELANOMA

*Not everything that is brown is a melanocytic tumor.*

*Not every melanocytic tumor is brown.*

---

**Box 1**
**Common benign lesions**

Melanocytic nevi

Skin tags

Seborrheic keratosis

Sebaceous hyperplasia

Syringoma

Epidermoid cysts

Dermatofibroma

Neurofibroma

Lipoma

Angioma

---

As the focus of this article is early identification, evaluation, and management of melanoma, a focus on pigmented lesions and melanocytic lesions is emphasized. Common benign "brown spots" on the face include solar lentigines, seborrheic keratosis, and melanocytic nevi. Dermatofibromas are often hyperpigmented as well, although they are rarely found on the face.

It is critically important to understand the distinction between "hypermelanosis" (normal number of melanocytes producing excess pigment) and melanocytic hyperplasia (proliferation of melanocytes, either benign, premalignant, or malignant). Furthermore, there are lesions associated with "hypomelanosis" and "amelanosis." The critical significance of this concept is clear when recognizing that the darkest pigmented seborrheic keratosis on the face is, in fact, not a melanocytic tumor at all but rather a benign proliferation of keratinocytes associated with dramatic hypermelanosis (ie, excess melanin from the normal benign melanocytes in the epidermis). Conversely, a deadly amelanotic nodular melanoma might present as a small pink nodule, yet histologically demonstrate a deep tumor of highly atypical melanocytic proliferation.

---

**Box 2**
**Common premalignant and malignant lesions**

Actinic keratosis

Dysplastic nevus

Basal cell carcinoma

Squamous cell carcinoma

Malignant melanoma

---

As with most malignancies, early detection is most critical. Fortunately, malignant lesions on high-risk patients can usually be caught early with ongoing and regular close monitoring. Furthermore, it is important to note the biology of different types of melanoma and to recognize that "early" and "late" correspond to biologic time rather than chronologic time. The most dramatic example would be a comparison between a rapidly growing nodular melanoma versus a typically indolent, slowly growing in situ lentigo maligna melanoma (LLM). In the first situation, it may be difficult to remove the tumor before it develops the potential for aggressive behavior even with optimal management. In the latter, it may be perfectly appropriate to observe and reevaluate for months or years before considering a biopsy (**Fig. 1**).

## SUBTYPES OF MELANOMA

- Superficial spreading melanoma (SSM)
- Nodular melanoma
- LLM
- Desmoplastic melanoma
- Acral lentiginous melanoma (palms and soles) (**Fig. 2**)

The identification of lesions suspicious for malignant melanoma rests on the clinician's ability to recognize all the possible clinical variations. This skill depends on clinician experience, history of the lesion, patient risk factors, and clinical morphology of the lesion.

Optimal biopsy of lesions suspicious for melanoma includes removal of the entire lesion for diagnosis and prognostic evaluation.[34] Although an excisional biopsy would no doubt provide this information, it is not always essential, and it may prove too time-consuming to be practical for the busy practitioner. In addition, the potential morbidity of a full-thickness excision (on the back, for example) is significant when compared with a scoop shave biopsy that can be performed quickly and managed with simple hemostasis and a adhesive bandage. Regarding biopsy on the face, it is important to note that in situ lesions can be removed for histologic evaluation with a very superficial shave just into the papillary dermis, and these superficial "abrasions" heal remarkably well by secondary intention. This is most relevant when evaluating for possible LLM, as discussed in detail later. Finally, an appropriate size punch biopsy can often remove the entire lesion in a very efficient fashion, and suture closure is typically straightforward. A skilled clinician should assess the risks and benefits of different biopsy

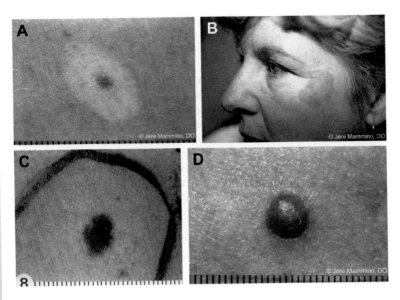

**Fig. 1.** Benign pigmented lesions. (*A*) Halo nevus, (*B*) solar lentigo, (*C*) atypical nevus, (*D*) dermatofibroma. (*Courtesy of* Jere J. Mammino, DO, FAAD, FAOCD, Maitland, FL)

techniques for each situation. It is important to note that biopsy technique does not affect ultimate prognosis. In summary, although excisional biopsy is preferred whenever possible, multiple biopsy techniques can be used to evaluate suspicious lesions, and the appropriate technique must be carefully selected based on clinical features.

A complete review and analysis of histopathologic features of melanoma are beyond the scope of this article, but several of the following fundamental findings should be addressed by the dermatopathologist:

a. Is this a melanocytic tumor?
b. Is the melanocytic proliferation histologically benign, malignant, or difficult to categorize ("dysplastic")?
c. signs of prognostic importance:
   • Breslow depth of invasion
   • Ulceration
   • Mitotic rate
   • Microsatellitosis
   • Histologic subtype
   • Regression
   • Neurotropism
   • Angiolymphatic and lymphovascular invasion

The most characteristic histologic findings of melanoma include atypical melanocytic hyperplasia at the dermoepidermal junction, with malignant melanocytes found individually and in nests. The nests of melanocytes can vary significantly in size, and individual malignant melanocytes typically scatter upward into all layers of the epidermis, so-called pagetoid spread. In invasive lesions, there is often an associated dermal inflammatory infiltrate and dermal melanophages. Not surprisingly, there are many patterns of melanocytic hyperplasia that create significant challenges in diagnosis, including both "recurrent benign nevi" and Spitz nevi.

In the absence of robust histologic and morphologic evidence to make a definitive diagnosis of melanoma, immunohistochemistry is an invaluable tool to confirm the melanocytic origin of the lesion.

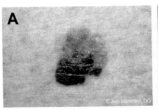 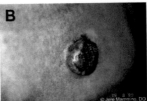 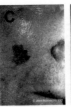 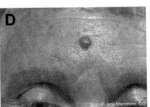

**Fig. 2.** Some types of melanoma that can present on the head and neck. (*A*) SSM, with characteristic "ABCDs of melanoma detection." (*B*) Nodular melanoma commonly grows more in thickness than in diameter. (*C*) LLM, varied pigmentation, ill-defined borders. (*D*) Desmoplastic melanoma, rare, often amelanotic form of melanoma. (*Courtesy of* Jere J. Mammino, DO, FAAD, FAOCD, Maitland, FL)

Sox10, S100, Melan-A/MART1, and HMB45 are some of the antibodies used to aid in the diagnoses, with Melan-A/MART1 and HMB45 offering the highest specificity of melanocytic differentiation.[35] In addition to morphology, histology, and immunohistochemistry, newer molecular diagnostic and prognostic tests are evolving and may further aid in management. Such tests include the fluorescence in situ hybridization diagnostic technique[36–38] and gene expression profiling.[39,40] However, currently, these techniques remain investigational and are not recommended for routine use.

## SUPERFICIAL SPREADING MELANOMA

SSM is the most common presentation for melanoma overall,[41–47] and it is typified by an initial often protracted "radial growth phase" where malignant melanocytic proliferation occurs radially on the surface of the skin preferentially to vertically into deeper layers of skin. Herein, the commonly cited "ABCDs" of melanoma are most pertinent in helping identify suspicious lesions. However, although most SSMs are associated with some or all of these well-known criteria, not all lesions demonstrating "ABCDs" are clinically suspicious. In fact, the likely most common lesions to demonstrate these features are common benign seborrheic keratosis.

## NODULAR MELANOMA

Fortunately, much less commonly, nodular melanoma is a form of melanoma with an aggressive vertical growth phase in the absence of a prominent radial growth phase. As such, Breslow thickness increases quickly over time along with metastatic potential. Although most lesions are pigmented, they can also be completely amelanotic and present as skin-colored or pink papules or nodules. With this challenging possibility, experienced clinicians should adhere to the basic tenet that any lesion that cannot be confidently given a benign clinical diagnosis could warrant a biopsy given the possibility of a relatively featureless amelanotic melanoma. Conversely, a clinician inexperienced in dermatologic evaluation may perform biopsies on an inordinate number of benign lesions because of their lack of familiarity with the vast lexicon of dermatologic pathology.

## LENTIGO MALIGNA MELANOMA

LLM most commonly presents on the head and neck, but it can present on other body locations.[48–52] Unique features include presentation on chronically sun-damaged skin, vague, ill-defined margins and very irregular shapes, and multiple shades of pigmentation. Histologically, atypical melanocytic hyperplasia is found at the basal layer of the epidermis extending down adnexal structures, and it can be difficult to determine the peripheral margins, as the malignant melanocytic hyperplasia gradually decreases at peripheral margins. For this reason, recurrences after standard excision are common,[53–57] and nonsurgical approaches can be considered as either primary or adjuvant therapy. Fortunately, the most important biologic feature of LMM is their tendency for indolent growth and low metastatic potential, with a prolonged radial growth phase that can span decades.[49,55,57–59] All these features combined make management of LMM particularly challenging.

## GUIDELINES OF CARE OF PRIMARY CUTANEOUS (HEAD AND NECK) MELANOMA

Once the diagnosis of melanoma is confirmed, staging is done using the American Joint Committee on Cancer TNM staging categories. Accurate staging is essential in guiding surgical and nonsurgical treatment, surveillance intensity, risk stratification, as well as other prognostic factors.[60–62] The staging of the primary tumor is based on histologic features of the initial skin biopsy (T1, 2, 3, 4a, and 4b). Sentinel lymph node biopsy (SLNB) has become the standard of care to define nodal staging. Although sentinel lymph node status is a powerful prognostic finding, the therapeutic role of SLNB is less well defined.[62–64] Finally, imaging studies are indicated only if the patient has signs or symptoms of metastatic disease.

Surgical removal of the primary tumor is done to ensure complete removal, complete histologic evaluation, and margin evaluation. It is also done to reduce local recurrence, although it has no impact on the risk for distant metastatic disease. Details of surgical management are provided in Pablo Nenclares and Kevin J Harrington's article, "Management of Head and Neck Mucosal Melanoma," in this issue.

In some situations, nonsurgical treatment of in situ LMM can be considered a reasonable option for first-line therapy or adjuvant therapy after surgery. The most well-studied topical therapy is imiquimod cream, an immune response modifier that often potentiates a brisk antitumor inflammatory response involving a broad expression of interferons and other cytokines. Several studies using imiquimod for the first-line treatment of in situ LMM report approximately 75% clinical and histologic clearance.[34,58,65] The use of adjuvant imiquimod after surgical excision has also been shown to be associated with a lower risk of recurrence. Although surgical excision is still considered optimal treatment for in situ LMM, topical imiquimod may be appropriate in select cases after careful consideration.[34] Finally, the use of radiation therapy in the treatment of melanoma in situ remains extremely uncommon in the United States.

All melanoma patients should have continued dermatologic follow-up for life to monitor for signs of recurrence as well as to detect new primary lesions.

## MULTIDISCIPLINARY APPROACH TO MELANOMA MANAGEMENT

Patients with early primary cutaneous melanoma (in situ and lesions less than 1 mm deep) can typically receive all appropriate care in the dermatologist's office, including initial skin examination, skin biopsy, patient consultation, and definitive excision. Deeper lesions with greater metastatic potential require coordinated care with pathologists, surgical oncologists, and medical oncologists. As diagnostic, prognostic, and therapeutic options for patients with advanced melanoma improve, a skilled team of melanoma specialists is optimal to coordinate the most effective strategies for each individual patient.

## CLINICS CARE POINTS

- When meeting a patient to evaluate a skin lesion, do not be in a hurry to examine the lesion before completing all other preliminary parts of the history. A specific lesion cannot be evaluated in a vacuum.

- When formulating a clinical differential diagnosis, try to knowledgeably formulate a clinicopathologic correlation.

- Carefully consider appropriate biopsy techniques based on anticipated clinicopathologic correlation.

- Always nurture an active professional relationship with your dermatopathologist and learn how mutual discussion can optimize best diagnosis and treatment.

## ACKNOWLEDGMENTS

All images in this article were obtained from Jere J. Mammino, DO, FAAD, FAOCD Program DirectorKCU-GMEC/Orlando Dermatology Residency Program.

## DISCLOSURE

The authors have no affiliations with or financial involvement in any organization or entity with a direct financial interest in the subject matter or materials discussed in the article.

## REFERENCES

1. Palamaras I, Semkova K. Perioperative management of and recommendations for antithrombotic medications in dermatological surgery. Br J Dermatol 2015;172(3):597–605.
2. Sporbeck B, Georges Bechara F, Häfner H-M, et al. S3 guidelines for the management of anticoagulation in cutaneous surgery. J Dtsch Dermatol Ges 2015;13(4):346–56.
3. Berríos-Torres SI, Umscheid CA, Bratzler DW, et al. Centers for Disease Control and Prevention guideline for the prevention of surgical site infection, 2017. JAMA Surg 2017;152(8):784.
4. Rosengren H, Dixon A. Antibacterial prophylaxis in dermatologic surgery: an evidence-based review. Am J Clin Dermatol 2010;11(1):35–44.
5. Johnson-Jahangir H, Agrawal N. Perioperative antibiotic use in cutaneous surgery. Dermatol Clin 2019;37(3):329–40.
6. Maragh SLH, Brown MD. Prospective evaluation of surgical site infection rate among patients with Mohs micrographic surgery without the use of prophylactic antibiotics. J Am Acad Dermatol 2008; 59(2):275–8.
7. The role of antibiotics in cutaneous surgery: overview, skin florae, prevention of infective endocarditis. Published online May 18, 2021. Available at: https://emedicine.medscape.com/article/1127413-overview#showall. [Accessed 24 May 2021].
8. Messingham MJ, Arpey CJ. Update on the use of antibiotics in cutaneous surgery. Dermatol Surg 2005;31(8 Pt 2):1068–78.
9. Fitzpatrick TB. "Soleil et peau". [Sun and skin]. Ournal Médecine Esthét Fr 1975;2:33–4.
10. Fitzpatrick TB. The validity and practicality of sun-reactive skin types I through VI. Arch Dermatol 1988;124(6):869–71.
11. Quevedo WC, Fitzpatrick TB, Pathak MA, et al. Role of light in human skin color variation. Am J Phys Anthropol 1975;43(3):393–408.
12. Ransohoff KJ, Jaju PD, Jaju PD, et al. Familial skin cancer syndromes: increased melanoma risk. J Am Acad Dermatol 2016;74(3):423–34. quiz 435–436.
13. Soura E, Eliades PJ, Shannon K, et al. Hereditary melanoma: update on syndromes and management: genetics of familial atypical multiple mole melanoma syndrome. J Am Acad Dermatol 2016;74(3):395–407. quiz 408–410.

14. Soura E, Eliades PJ, Shannon K, et al. Hereditary melanoma: update on syndromes and management: emerging melanoma cancer complexes and genetic counseling. J Am Acad Dermatol 2016;74(3):411–20. quiz 421–422.

15. Christodoulou E, Nell RJ, Verdijk RM, et al. Loss of wild-type CDKN2A is an early event in the development of melanoma in FAMMM syndrome. J Invest Dermatol 2020;140(11):2298–301.e3.

16. Toussi A, Mans N, Welborn J, et al. Germline mutations predisposing to melanoma. J Cutan Pathol 2020;47(7):606–16.

17. Liu MT, Liu JY, Su J. CDKN2A gene in melanoma. Zhonghua Bing Li Xue Za Zhi 2019;48(11):909–12.

18. Read J, Wadt KAW, Hayward NK. Melanoma genetics. J Med Genet 2016;53(1):1–14.

19. Katsambas A, Nicolaidou E. Cutaneous malignant melanoma and sun exposure. Recent developments in epidemiology. Arch Dermatol 1996;132(4):444–50.

20. Elwood JM. Melanoma and sun exposure. Semin Oncol 1996;23(6):650–66.

21. Gandini S, Sera F, Cattaruzza MS, et al. Meta-analysis of risk factors for cutaneous melanoma: II. Sun exposure. Eur J Cancer 2005;41(1):45–60.

22. Pfahlberg A, Kölmel KF, Gefeller O, Febim Study Group. Timing of excessive ultraviolet radiation and melanoma: epidemiology does not support the existence of a critical period of high susceptibility to solar ultraviolet radiation- induced melanoma. Br J Dermatol 2001;144(3):471–5.

23. Westerdahl J, Olsson H, Ingvar C. At what age do sunburn episodes play a crucial role for the development of malignant melanoma. Eur J Cancer 1994;30A(11):1647–54.

24. Dennis LK, Vanbeek MJ, Beane Freeman LE, et al. Sunburns and risk of cutaneous melanoma: does age matter? A comprehensive meta-analysis. Ann Epidemiol 2008;18(8):614–27.

25. El Ghissassi F, Baan R, Straif K, et al. A review of human carcinogens—part D: radiation. Lancet Oncol 2009;10(8):751–2.

26. Ferrucci LM, Cartmel B, Molinaro AM, et al. Indoor tanning and risk of early-onset basal cell carcinoma. J Am Acad Dermatol 2012;67(4):552–62.

27. The association of use of sunbeds with cutaneous malignant melanoma and other skin cancers: a systematic review. Int J Cancer 2007;120(5):1116–22.

28. Watson M, Holman DM, Fox KA, et al. Preventing skin cancer through reduction of indoor tanning. Am J Prev Med 2013;44(6):682–9.

29. Lazovich D, Vogel RI, Berwick M, et al. Indoor tanning and risk of melanoma: a case-control study in a highly exposed population. Cancer Epidemiol Biomarkers Prev 2010;19(6):1557–68.

30. Rosa DF, Sarandy MM, Novaes RD, et al. High-fat diet and alcohol intake promotes inflammation and impairs skin wound healing in Wistar rats. Mediators Inflamm 2018;2018:4658583.

31. Goodman GD, Kaufman J, Day D, et al. Impact of smoking and alcohol use on facial aging in women: results of a large multinational, multiracial, cross-sectional survey. J Clin Aesthet Dermatol 2019; 12(8):28–39.

32. Dores GM, Huycke MM, Devesa SS. Melanoma of the skin and laterality. J Am Acad Dermatol 2011; 64(1):193–5.

33. Butler ST, Fosko SW. Increased prevalence of left-sided skin cancers. J Am Acad Dermatol 2010; 63(6):1006–10.

34. Swetter SM, Tsao H, Bichakjian CK, et al. Guidelines of care for the management of primary cutaneous melanoma. J Am Acad Dermatol 2019;80(1):208–50.

35. Kim RH, Meehan SA. Immunostain use in the diagnosis of melanomas referred to a tertiary medical center: a 15-year retrospective review (2001-2015). J Cutan Pathol 2017;44(3):221–7.

36. Gerami P, Li G, Pouryazdanparast P, et al. A highly specific and discriminatory FISH assay for distinguishing between benign and malignant melanocytic neoplasms. Am J Surg Pathol 2012;36(6):808–17.

37. Fang Y, Dusza S, Jhanwar S, et al. Fluorescence in situ hybridization (FISH) analysis of melanocytic nevi and melanomas: sensitivity, specificity, and lack of association with sentinel node status. Int J Surg Pathol 2012;20(5):434–40.

38. Gerami P, Jewell SS, Morrison LE, et al. Fluorescence in situ hybridization (FISH) as an ancillary diagnostic tool in the diagnosis of melanoma. Am J Surg Pathol 2009;33(8):1146–56.

39. Clarke LE, Warf MB, Flake DD, et al. Clinical validation of a gene expression signature that differentiates benign nevi from malignant melanoma. J Cutan Pathol 2015;42(4):244–52.

40. Clarke LE, Flake DD, Busam K, et al. An independent validation of a gene expression signature to differentiate malignant melanoma from benign melanocytic nevi. Cancer 2017;123(4):617–28.

41. Minini R, Rohrmann S, Braun R, et al. Incidence trends and clinical-pathological characteristics of invasive cutaneous melanoma from 1980 to 2010 in the Canton of Zurich, Switzerland. Melanoma Res 2017;27(2):145–51.

42. Singh P, Kim HJ, Schwartz RA. Superficial spreading melanoma: an analysis of 97702 cases using the SEER database. Melanoma Res 2016;26(4):395–400.

43. Allan BJ, Ovadia S, Tashiro J, et al. Superficial spreading melanomas in children: an analysis of outcomes using the Surveillance, Epidemiology, and End Results (SEER) database. Ann Plast Surg 2015;75(3):327–31.

44. Elder DE, Bastian BC, Cree IA, et al. The 2018 World Health Organization classification of cutaneous,

mucosal, and uveal melanoma: detailed analysis of 9 distinct subtypes defined by their evolutionary pathway. Arch Pathol Lab Med 2020;144(4):500–22.

45. Bobos M. Histopathologic classification and prognostic factors of melanoma: a 2020 update. Ital J Dermatol Venereol 2021;156(3):300–21.

46. McGovern VJ. The classification of melanoma and its relationship with prognosis. Pathology (Phila) 1970;2(2):85–98.

47. Rastrelli M, Tropea S, Rossi CR, et al. Melanoma: epidemiology, risk factors, pathogenesis, diagnosis and classification. In Vivo 2014;28(6):1005–11.

48. Matas-Nadal C, Malvehy J, Ferreres JR, et al. Increasing incidence of lentigo maligna and lentigo maligna melanoma in Catalonia. Int J Dermatol 2019;58(5):577–81.

49. Situm M, Bolanca Z, Buljan M. Lentigo maligna melanoma–the review. Coll Antropol 2010;34(Suppl 2): 299–301.

50. Ding Y, Jiang R, Chen Y, et al. Comparing the characteristics and predicting the survival of patients with head and neck melanoma versus body melanoma: a population-based study. BMC Cancer 2021;21(1):420.

51. Iznardo H, Garcia-Melendo C, Yélamos O. Lentigo maligna: clinical presentation and appropriate management. Clin Cosmet Investig Dermatol 2020;13: 837–55.

52. Wee E, Wolfe R, Mclean C, et al. The anatomic distribution of cutaneous melanoma: a detailed study of 5141 lesions. Australas J Dermatol 2020;61(2): 125–33.

53. Osborne JE, Hutchinson PE. A follow-up study to investigate the efficacy of initial treatment of lentigo maligna with surgical excision. Br J Plast Surg 2002;55(8):611–5.

54. DeBloom JR, Zitelli JA, Brodland DG. The invasive growth potential of residual melanoma and melanoma in situ. Dermatol Surg 2010;36(8):1251–7.

55. Kasprzak JM, Xu YG. Diagnosis and management of lentigo maligna: a review. Drugs Context 2015;4:212281.

56. Ren M, Kong YY, Shen XX, et al. Lentigo maligna and lentigo maligna melanoma: a clinicopathologic analysis of twenty-four cases. Zhonghua Bing Li Xue Za Zhi 2018;47(10):769–74.

57. Fröhlich SM, Cazzaniga S, Kaufmann LS, et al. A retrospective cohort study on patients with lentigo maligna melanoma. Dermatol Basel Switz 2019;235(4): 340–5.

58. Stevenson O, Ahmed I. Lentigo maligna: prognosis and treatment options. Am J Clin Dermatol 2005; 6(3):151–64.

59. Sina N, Saeed-Kamil Z, Ghazarian D. Pitfalls in the diagnosis of lentigo maligna and lentigo maligna melanoma, facts and an opinion. J Clin Pathol 2021;74(1):7–9.

60. Amin MB, Edge S, Greene F, et al, editors. AJCC cancer staging manual. 8th edition. Manhattan (NY): Springer International Publishing; 2017.

61. Gershenwald JE, Scolyer RA, Hess KR, et al. Melanoma staging: evidence-based changes in the American Joint Committee on Cancer eighth edition cancer staging manual. CA Cancer J Clin 2017;67(6):472–92.

62. Morrison S, Han D. Re-evaluation of sentinel lymph node biopsy for melanoma. Curr Treat Options Oncol 2021;22(3):22.

63. McMasters KM, Egger ME, Edwards MJ, et al. Final results of the sunbelt melanoma trial: a multi-institutional prospective randomized phase III study evaluating the role of adjuvant high-dose interferon alfa-2b and completion lymph node dissection for patients staged by sentinel lymph node biopsy. J Clin Oncol 2016;34(10):1079–86.

64. Morton DL, Thompson JF, Cochran AJ, et al. Final trial report of sentinel-node biopsy versus nodal observation in melanoma. N Engl J Med 2014;370(7):599–609.

65. Spenny ML, Walford J, Werchniak AE, et al. Lentigo maligna (melanoma in situ) treated with imiquimod cream 5%: 12 case reports. Cutis 2007;79(2):149–52.

# Classification and Staging of Melanoma in the Head and Neck

Anthony M. Bunnell, MD, DMD*, Stacey M. Nedrud, MD, DMD,
Rui P. Fernandes, MD, DMD, FRCS (Ed)

## KEYWORDS

- Cutaneous melanoma • Head and neck melanoma • AJCC Staging • Breslow thickness
- Ulceration • Melanoma prognosis • Maxillofacial surgery

## KEY POINTS

- The skin of the head and neck accounts for 18 to 22% of all melanomas, with the scalp and cheeks being the most common areas involved.
- Prognostic data for staging purposes are based on the more common subtypes (superficial spreading and nodular melanoma) as defined by the AJCC and World Health Organization
- Tumor thickness (Breslow thickness) and ulceration are 2 independent prognostic factors that have been shown to be the strongest predictors of survival and outcome.
- Clark level of invasion and mitotic rate are no longer incorporated into the current AJCC staging system, but still have shown to be important prognostic factors for cutaneous melanoma.
- LDH has been shown to be an independent predictor of survival outcome among patients with metastatic (Stage IV) disease

## INTRODUCTION

According to the American Cancer Society, the rates of melanoma have continued to rise over the past few decades. Recent estimates have shown that 18% to 22% of new melanoma cases occur within the head and neck in the United States each year.[1] The most common sites within the head and neck are the occipital scalp and skin of the cheek. The mainstay of the treatment of nonmetastatic primary melanomas of the head and neck includes surgical resection and management of regional disease as indicated, but management strategies for advanced systemic disease have progressed significantly with the introduction of checkpoint inhibitor immunotherapy and molecular targeted therapy. Since the introduction of Ipilimumab in 2011, 9 new therapies have been approved for unresectable melanoma, along with 4 new approvals in the adjuvant

therapy setting.[2] While the incidence of melanoma continues to increase over the past 30 years, overall survival has also been improving with the advent of these new therapies[3] Knowledge of the classification and staging of melanoma is critical to provide the standard of care to these patients. The Maxillofacial surgeon must remain apprised of the most current management strategies in this patient population. Classification systems and staging provide the foundation for clinical decision making and prognostication for the maxillofacial surgeon when caring for these patients.

## MELANOMA SUBTYPES AND CLASSIFICATION

The classification of the various subtypes of melanoma has undergone significant transformation as the initial classification schemes first introduced by McGovern[4] and Clark[5]. Since then, advances

Division of Head and Neck Surgery, Department of Oral and Maxillofacial Surgery, University of Florida College of Medicine,- Jacksonville 653-1 West 8th, Street, Jacksonville, FL 32209, USA
* Corresponding author.
E-mail address: anthony.bunnell@jax.ufl.edu

Oral Maxillofacial Surg Clin N Am 34 (2022) 221–234
https://doi.org/10.1016/j.coms.2021.12.001
1042-3699/22/© 2021 Elsevier Inc. All rights reserved.

in the understanding of the biological behavior, histopathology, and genetic origins of melanoma have allowed for the development and progression of additional classification systems. The World Health Organization Classification of Skin Tumors 4th edition provides a classification system based on epidemiology, clinical and histologic morphology, and genomic characteristics[6]. Melanoma is classified based on the site of origin (epithelium-associated vs nonepithelium associated), mole phenotype (high vs low nevus count), frequency of BRAF, NRAS, and other relevant mutations. Cutaneous melanoma is divided into 2 groups; those related to sun exposure and those not related to sun exposure. This is based on the consideration that solar damage is one of the main causative factors of cutaneous melanoma. These 2 groups are then further divided, based on the degree of sun exposure, into low and high cumulative solar damage groups. **Table 1** highlights the main classification groups in the 4th edition of the World Health Organization Classification of Skin Tumors.

The traditional clinicopathologic classification of melanoma is based on morphologic aspects of the growth phase and distinguishes 4 main subtypes as defined by the World Health Organization: superficial spreading, nodular, acral lentiginous, and lentigo-maligna melanoma.

Characteristics of each of these subtypes are further described in **Table 2**. Other less common subtypes have also been described, including amelanotic and desmoplastic melanoma.

Desmoplastic is a variant of interest due to its improved disease-specific survival, despite an often delay in diagnosis due to its amelanotic appearance. According to the 8th edition of the AJCC Staging Manual, the data used to derive the TNM Categories were based largely on superficial spreading melanoma and nodular subtypes.

Despite some differences in etiology and pathogenesis within various subtypes, the AJCC recommends the same staging criteria be used for melanomas with any growth pattern.

## GENETIC CHARACTERIZATION OF MELANOMA

Melanoma is one of the most highly mutated malignancies, mainly as a function of its generation through ultraviolet light and other mutational processes. The vast number of mutations provides an overwhelming and often confusing amount of data, even more so with recent advances in targeted and immune therapy. While mutations in BRAF V6000 are known to display sensitivity to BRAF and mitogen-activated protein kinase (MEK) inhibitors, the clinical implications and prognostic value of the other mutations are far less understood and are beyond the scope of this article. Advances in multiple molecular genetic techniques including polymerase chain reaction (PCR), massively parallel sequencing (next-generation sequencing), fluorescence in situ hybridization (FISH), and comparative genomic hybridization have recognized that several chromosomal aberrations and genetic mutations can assist with the diagnosis and management of melanoma[13] Next-generation sequencing has allowed for the sequencing of multiple oncogenes implicated in melanoma (BRAF, NRAS, PREX2, GRIN2A, ERBB4) in a single assessment as a first step toward personalized medicine.[14] While gene expression profiling has been used for uveal melanoma, it may have extended applicability with some studies showing improved diagnostic and prognostic utility[2,15] but this remains controversial for use in cutaneous melanoma staging at this time.[16,17] Gene expression profiling has been incorporated into consensus guidelines by the

---

**Table 1**
**WHO classification of melanoma 2018**

| | |
|---|---|
| Melanomas Associated with Cumulative Solar Damage (CSD)[a] | Superficial Spreading Melanoma<br>Lentigo Maligna Melanoma<br>Desmoplastic Melanoma |
| Melanomas not associated with cumulative solar damage (CSD)[a] | Spitz melanomas<br>Acral melanoma<br>Mucosal melanomas<br>Melanomas arising in congenital nevi<br>Melanomas arising in blue nevi<br>Uveal melanoma |

[a] WHO classification system states that nodular melanoma may occur in any or most of the above subtypes.
*From* Bastian BC, de la Fouchardiere A, Elder DE, et al. Genomic landscape of melanoma. In: Elder DE, Massi D, Scolyer RA, Willemze R, eds. WHO Classification of Skin Tumours. 4th ed. Lyon, France: IARC; 2018:72–75. World Health Organization Classification of Tumours; vol 11.

**Table 2**
**Morphologic classification of melanoma subtypes**

| Melanoma Subtype | Frequency | Common Features Associated with Each Subtype | Site Predilection (if Applicable) |
|---|---|---|---|
| Superficial Spreading | • Most common subtype<br>• 70%–75% of all melanomas[7] | • Over 60% are thin $\leq$ 1 mm thickness<br>• Characteristic horizontal growth pattern<br>• Subtype most likely to be associated with a pre-existing nevus.<br>• Highly curable | • All sites<br>• Lower extremities in women |
| Nodular | • Second most common type<br>• 15%–30% of all melanomas | • Most are thicker than 2 mm at the time of diagnoses[8]<br>• Appear as darkly pigmented, pedunculated, or polypoid papules or nodules<br>• Early detection can be difficult and often invasive at presentation[8] | • Extremities and trunk<br>• Scalp (most common site in head and neck) |
| Acral Lentiginous | • < 5% of all melanomas | • More common in African Americans and Asians<br>• Clinically appear as irregularly pigmented macules or patches (dark brown to black)[9] | • Palmar and Plantar Surfaces<br>• Subungual (in the nail beds) Surfaces |
| Lentigo Maligna | • 10%–15% of all melanomas | • More common in chronic sun-damaged areas in older individuals<br>• Clinically begins as a freckle-like, tan-brown macule[10] | • Any sun-exposed area |
| Amelanotic Melanoma | • 2%–10% of all melanomas[11] | Clinical appearance mistaken for other benign lesions (dermal nevus, inflamed seborrheic keratosis, hemangioma) | • All sites |
| Desmoplastic Melanoma | • < 4% of all melanomas | • Appears as a slowly growing plaque, nodule, or scar-like growth<br>• Early diagnoses challenging due to amelanotic appearance<br>• Delay in diagnosis can lead to thicker tumor at the time of diagnosis[12] | • Chronic sun-exposed areas in older individuals |

Melanoma Prevention Working Group and the National Comprehensive Cancer Network but it is not currently used in the current AJCC staging guidelines.[16,18]

## CLINICAL CLASSIFICATION AND STAGING

Melanoma is diagnosed histopathologically following initial biopsy, which will assist with classifying the tumor to guide treatment. Classification is based on tumor thickness and ulceration (T stage, Breslow Staging), Regional Lymph Node Involvement (N Stage), and presence of metastasis (M Stage).

Clinical staging is based on information obtained from:

- The initial biopsy of the primary melanoma (including microstaging)
- Clinical or biopsy assessment of regional lymph nodes

Pathologic staging is based on information obtained from:

- The initial biopsy of the primary melanoma
- Wide local excision of the primary melanoma
- Pathological evaluation of the regional lymph node basin obtained from either:
  - Sentinel lymph node biopsy (required for N categorization of all > T1 melanomas)
  - Complete regional lymphadenectomy

## PRIMARY TUMOR STAGING

In the United States, recent estimates have shown that 84% of patients with melanoma (all sites) initially present with localized disease, 9% with regional disease, and 4% with distant metastatic disease.[19] In patients with localized disease and primary tumors 1.0 mm or less in thickness, 5-year survival is reached by more than 90% of patients. Once tumor thickness increases greater than 1.0 mm, survival rates vary considerably from 50% to 90% depending on tumor thickness, ulceration, and mitotic rate.[20]

Tumor thickness and ulceration remain the 2 main criteria for determining the T category. The T category is divided into T1–T4 based on the tumor thickness. Each category is further subdivided into a and b, delineated by the absence or presence of ulceration, respectively. *Melanoma in situ* that was previously under Stage 0 category, is now categorized as Tis. T0 is now reserved for patients with no evidence of primary tumor.

## BRESLOW THICKNESS

The T category is defined primarily by measuring the thickness of the tumor. This is classically described by Alexander Breslow,[21] who reported that tumor thickness is the most crucial criteria for prognostication and management. Breslow thickness has been shown to be the most consistently reproducible factor in melanoma histopathology reporting.[22] To that end, the AJCC 8th edition has clarified how tumor thickness should

be recorded to ensure consistency and reproducibility among pathologists. Currently, the AJCC recommends that tumor thickness are measured from the top of the granular layer to the deepest invasive cell across the broad base of the tumor (**Fig. 1**). The thickness measurement should be recorded to the nearest 0.1 mm, previously 0.01 mm, changed due to impracticality and imprecision of measurements.[22] T category thresholds of melanoma thickness continue to be defined in whole number integers (1.0, 2.0, and 4.0 mm). For example, T2 category is now reflected as 1.0 to 2.0 mm (as opposed to 1.01–2.0 mm in the 7th edition) and is illustrated in **Table 3**.

Multiple reports in the literature have shown that survival in patients with a T1 melanoma is related to tumor thickness, with a possible clinically important "breakpoint" in the region of 0.7 to 0.8 mm [20,21,23–25] A multivariate analysis looked at several prognostic factors including 0.8 mm tumor thickness threshold, mitotic rate and ulceration, and their effect on melanoma-specific survival among patients with a T1 melanoma. Tumor thickness (dichotomized into 2 groups <0.8 mm and 0.8–1.0 mm) and ulceration were shown to be stronger predictors of melanoma-specific survival than mitotic rate. The 8th edition of the AJCC staging manual has since removed tumor mitotic rate as a staging criterion for T1 tumors, but the AJCC still recommends that it remains an important prognostic factor and should continue to be recorded. This tumor thickness threshold of 0.8 mm is reflected in the T1 categorization:

- T1a: nonulcerated, less than 0.8 mm in thickness

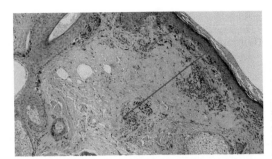

**Fig. 1.** T1a melanoma. Invasive melanoma that measures less than 0.8 mm in thickness without ulceration. Tumor thickness (Breslow thickness) is measured from the top of the granular layer to the deepest invasive cell across the broad base of the tumor. (*Courtesy of* Ibraheem Javeed Mohammed and Reeba Omman, MDs, Gainesville, FL)

| Table 3 American Joint Committee on Cancer Eighth Edition: T category for Cutaneous Melanoma | | |
|---|---|---|
| **T Category** | **T Criteria** | |
| TX: | Primary tumor thickness cannot be assessed (eg, diagnosis by curettage) | |
| T0: | No evidence of primary tumor (eg, unknown primary or completely regressed melanoma) | |
| Tis | Melanoma in situ | |
| | **Thickness** | **Ulceration status** |
| T1 | ≤1.0 mm | Unknown or unspecified |
| T1a | <0.8 mm | Without ulceration |
| T1b | <0.8 mm 0.8–1 mm | With ulceration With or without ulceration |
| T2 | >1–2 mm | Unknown or unspecified |
| T2a | >1–2 mm | Without ulceration |
| T2b | >1–2 mm | With ulceration |
| T3 | >2–4 mm | Unknown or unspecified |
| T3a | >2–4 mm | Without ulceration |
| T3b | >2–4 mm | With ulceration |
| T4 | >4 mm | Unknown or unspecified |
| T4a | >4 mm | Without ulceration |
| T4b | >4 mm | With ulceration |

Data from Gershenwald JE, Scolyer RA, Hess KR, et al. Melanoma of the skin. In: Amin MB, Edge SB, Greene FL, et al, eds. AJCC Cancer Staging Manual. 7th and 8th eds. New York: Springer International Publishing; 2010 and 2017.

- T1b defined as 0.8 to 1.0 mm in thickness (regardless of ulceration) OR ulcerated melanomas 0.8 mm in thickness.

This 0.8 mm thickness threshold has clinical implications in decision making for the role of sentinel lymph node biopsy in patients with T1 melanomas. Several studies have shown there is a low rate of sentinel lymph node metastasis (<5%) in tumors less than 0.8 mm in thickness, whereas rates of sentinel lymph node metastases approach 5% to 12% in patients with tumors 0.8 to 1.0 mm in thickness.[26–29] It is, for this reason, that guideline recommendations suggest that sentinel lymph node biopsy should be considered for tumors 0.8 to 1.0 mm in thickness, especially in the presence of other adverse factors. This will be discussed in-depth within another article in this edition.

## ULCERATION

Ulceration has been shown to be an independent advanced prognostic factor in primary cutaneous melanoma.[20,30–32] Outcomes are worse for patients with ulcerated primary melanomas than compared with those patients with nonulcerated primary melanomas of the same thickness.[33,34] As previously mentioned, ulceration is considered the second major criteria for the determination of T stage category. Ulceration is defined as a combination of the following features:

- Full-thickness epidermal defect (including the absence of stratum corneum and basement membrane of the dermo-epidermal junction
- Evidence of reactive changes (fibrin deposition, neutrophils)
- Thinning, effacement, or reactive hyperplasia of the surrounding epidermis in the absence of trauma or a recent surgical procedure

These features can assist pathologists when a lesion has recently been biopsied or there is difficulty determining if epidermal dehiscence is due to ulceration or sectioning artifact. The lack of neutrophils and fibrin deposition are likely then due to sectioning artifact rather than true ulceration. The AJCC recommends the following regarding ulceration:

- Epidermal loss caused by a prior biopsy should not be recorded as ulceration for staging purposes
- Nontraumatic ulceration that is present should be recorded as ulceration for staging purposes
- Ulceration is reported as either unknown, present, or absent within the T category

If ulceration is present, the measurement is taken from the base of the ulcer to the broadest base of the tumor (**Fig. 2**). This is subcategorized as T staging criteria and listed accordingly in **Table 3**.

## MITOTIC RATE

As previously mentioned, the mitotic rate was removed as staging criterion in the most recent 8th edition of the AJCC staging system because substratifying T1 tumors using the 0.8 mm tumor thickness threshold and the presence or absence of ulceration showed stronger associations with outcome. Despite this, the mitotic rate remains a major determinant of prognosis for melanomas of all thickness categories. A recent systematic review and meta-analysis established that the presence of mitoses was the most important predictor

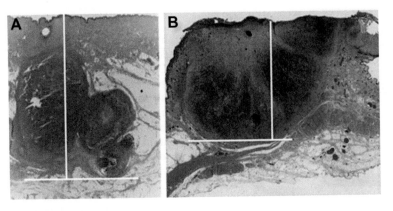

**Fig. 2.** (*A*) T4a melanoma – Measuring greater than 4.0 mm in thickness. Measured from the top of the granular layer of the intact epidermis to the deepest invasive cell across the broad base of the tumor. (*B*) T4b melanoma - Measuring greater than 4.0 mm in thickness with ulcerated epithelium. Tumor thickness is measured from the base of the ulcer to the deepest invasive cell across the broad base of the tumor. (*Courtesy of* Ibraheem Javeed Mohammed and Reeba Omman, MDs, Gainesville, FL)

of sentinel lymph node metastases in primary thin melanomas.[35,36] To that end, the AJCC still recommends mitotic rate be recorded for all patients with T1–T4 primary cutaneous melanoma to assist with future prognostic data analysis.

## CLARK LEVEL OF INVASION

Historically, Breslow thickness and Clark's level of invasion were the 2 methods used to measure depth and level of invasion to assist with the staging of the primary tumor. Clark's level of invasion is based on anatomic layers of the skin that the tumor has invaded. For descriptive purposes, Clark's level of invasion is described in **Table 4**. Clark's level is less reproducible than tumor thickness among pathologist due to limitations in interpreting differences between the papillary and reticular dermis in patients with solar elastosis or in certain areas such as the scalp. Historically,

Clark's level of invasion was used to describe the specific subcategory of thin T1 melanomas in the AJCC 6th edition; it has since been removed due to low statistical correlation with survival compared with 6 independent prognostic variables in the 7th edition of the AJCC Staging Manual 7th edition.[20] While Clark's Level of invasion has been removed from the 7th edition, multiple analyses have shown Clark's levels to be an independent prognostic factor.[37] The AJCC still recommends it should be recorded as a primary tumor characteristic.

## STAGING OF REGIONAL LYMPH NODES

As stated earlier, the management of regional and systemic disease has evolved significantly over the past 2 decades. It is known that the presence of lymph node metastasis carries a major prognostic implication; therefore, detection of occult metastasis is crucial for accurate staging.[38–40] Among patients with nodal metastasis (Stage III), the clinical nodal status (nonpalpable vs palpable) and the number of metastatic nodes are the most important predictors of survival.[41,42] The 8th edition of the AJCC staging manual has recognized the difference in prognosis among patients with pathologic Stage III Melanoma (any ≥ N1).[20] Regional lymph node involvement is described as either clinically occult metastasis detected via microscopic evaluation from sentinel lymph node biopsy, or clinically detected metastasis to regional lymph nodes. Clinical detection is through either physical examination, ultrasound, computed tomography (CT), or positron emission tomography (PET/CT). In the absence of signs and symptoms that may suggest disease spread, selective use of CT or PET/CT based on clinical stage may identify occult metastases and result in more accurate stage determination.[43]

| Table 4 Clark's level of invasion | |
|---|---|
| Level I | Melanoma Confined to the Epidermis (melanoma in Situ) |
| Level II | Melanoma cells invade into, but do not fill or expand, the papillary (superficial) dermis |
| Level III | Melanoma cells fill and expand the papillary dermis with the extension of tumor to the papillary-reticular dermal interface |
| Level IV | Melanoma cells infiltrate into the reticular dermis |
| Level V | Melanoma cells infiltrate into the subcutaneous fat |

Clinically occult regional lymph node disease is typically detected by lymphatic mapping (lymphoscintigraphy) and sentinel lymph node biopsy, the indications for which will be discussed further in this issue. These patients with clinically occult disease were previously defined as having microscopic disease in the 7th edition. These clinically occult patients represent a vast majority of the overall patients who present with regional metastasis at the time of diagnosis. Patients with clinically occult nodal disease are categorized into N1a, N2a, or N3a based on the number of involved nodes, unless nonnodal locoregional disease is present (microsatellites, satellites, or in-transit metastases). These are also referred to as intralymphatic regional metastases and have been shown to be associated with a poor prognosis.[44,45]

*Microsatellites* are defined as microscopic cutaneous or subcutaneous metastases that are adjacent to or just deep to the primary tumor noted on histopathological analysis. By definition, these metastatic tumor cells must be discontinuous from the primary tumor. The College of American Pathologists define a microsatellite as the presence of tumor nests greater than 0.05 mm in diameter, located within the reticular dermis, panniculus, or vessels beneath the principle invasive tumor but separated from it by at least 0.3 mm of normal tissue.[46] The 8th edition of the AJCC Staging Manual defines a microsatellite as a microscopic cutaneous or subcutaneous metastasis adjacent to, or deep to, and completely discontinuous from a primary melanoma with unaffected stroma occupying the space between, identified on the pathological examination of the primary tumor site.[32] Satellite metastases are defined as any focus or clinically evident cutaneous or subcutaneous metastases occurring within 2 cm of, but discontinuous from, the primary melanoma. In-transit metastases are defined as clinically evident cutaneous or subcutaneous metastases occurring >2 cm from the primary melanoma in the region between the primary and the regional lymph nodes. Patients with any of the 3 (microsatellite, satellite, or in-transit metastases) are staged N1c, N2c, or N3c (**Table 5**) according to the number of involved nodes, regardless of whether they are clinically occult or clinically detected.

Clinically evident nodal disease is categorized into N1b, N2b, or N3b based on the number of involved lymph nodes. If one node is detected clinically and additional nodes are then detected during microscopic examination (those noted only on microscopic examination following lymphadenectomy), the total number of lymph nodes should be recorded for N categorization. The 8th edition of the AJCC removed the term "gross nodal extension" as an N category criteria. Matted nodes (2 or more nodes adherent to one another through involvement by metastatic disease) are still used within the N3 category. The AJCC still recommends recording the presence of extranodal extension following histopathologic analysis, but this is not currently used for staging purposes.

## DISTANT METASTASIS

Melanoma has the potential to metastasize to any organ or site. Common sites for metastasis include skin, subcutaneous tissue, lymph nodes, lungs, liver, brain, and visceral organs. Metastases typically occur within a few years following the initial diagnosis. Late metastasis (decades later) is far less common for cutaneous melanoma. For patients with metastatic disease, the following anatomic sites of distant metastasis are used to define the M categories into four subcategories:

- *M1a:* Skin, soft tissue, including muscle, and or nonregional lymph node
- *M1b:* Lung
- *M1c:* Non-CNS visceral sites
- *M1d:* CNS

The site of metastasis is known to be the most significant predictor of outcome. As expected, M1a portends a relatively better prognosis compared with any of the other anatomic sites. M1b prognosis is described as "intermediate." M1c now includes only non-CNS visceral sites in the new edition and has a worse prognosis than patients within the M1b category. For patients with CNS metastasis, a separate M1d category was added to the 8th edition. M1d has the worst prognosis of any of the M categories. Serum Lactate Dehydrogenase (LDH) is a well-known biomarker for patients with metastatic melanoma and has been part of the AJCC staging guidelines since 2009.[47] LDH has been shown to be an independent predictor of survival outcome among patients with Stage IV disease.[48–51] More recent trials involving immune checkpoint inhibitors have shown that elevated LDH levels are associated with poor survival and poor response rates.[52,53] A retrospective study reported that increases in LDH levels between the start of treatment and the first staging were associated with poor response and diminished overall survival in patients receiving the PD-1 antibodies Nivolumab or Pembrolizumab.[54] Previously, patients with metastatic disease to any site with an elevated serum LDH were placed into the high-risk category M1c.[20] Serum LDH is now used to define each M

**Table 5**
**American Joint Committee on Cancer Eighth Edition: N category for Cutaneous Melanoma**

| N Category | N Criteria<br>Number of Tumor-Involved Regional Lymph Nodes | Presence of In-transit, Satellite, And/Or Microsatellite Metastases |
|---|---|---|
| NX | Regional nodes not assessed (eg, SLN biopsy not performed, regional nodes previously removed for another reason)<br>Exception: Pathologic N category is not required for T1 melanomas, use cN | No |
| N0 | No regional metastases detected | No |
| N1 | One tumor-involved node or in-transit, satellite, and/or microsatellite metastases with no tumor-involved nodes | Yes |
| N1a | One clinically occult node (ie, detected by SLN biopsy) | No |
| N1b | One clinically detected node | No |
| N1c | No regional lymph node disease | Yes |
| N2 | Two or three tumor-involved nodes or in-transit, satellite, and/or microsatellite metastases with one tumor-involved node | Yes |
| N2a | Two or 3 clinically occult (ie, detected by SLN biopsy) | No |
| N2b | Two or 3, at least one of which was clinically detected | No |
| N2c | One clinically occult or clinically detected | Yes |
| N3 | Four or more tumor-involved nodes or in-transit, satellite, and/or microsatellite metastases with 2 or more tumor-involved nodes, or any number of matted nodes without or with in-transit, satellite, and/or microsatellite metastases | Yes |
| N3a | Four or more clinically occult (ie, detected by SLN biopsy) | No |
| N3b | Four or more, at least one of which was clinically detected, or presence of any number of matted nodes | No |
| N3c | Two or more clinically occult or clinically detected and/or presence of any number of matted nodes | Yes |

*Data from* Gershenwald JE, Scolyer RA, Hess KR, et al. Melanoma of the skin. In: Amin MB, Edge SB, Greene FL, et al, eds. AJCC Cancer Staging Manual. 7th and 8th eds. New York: Springer International Publishing; 2010 and 2017.

category in the 8th edition and further illustrated in **Table 6**.

## THE ROLE OF IMAGING FOR STAGE DETERMINATION

The role of imaging will be briefly reviewed here, as indications for imaging will be discussed within another section of this edition. T Category staging for melanoma of all stages is largely predicated on histologic confirmation rather than radiographic evaluation. Radiographic imaging is more often used for refining clinical staging by detecting the presence of regional or distant disease. According to the NCCN Melanoma Guidelines,[18] imaging is not typically indicated for thin, low-risk melanomas (pT1a). Other Imaging modalities to be considered for the remaining stages include ultrasound to evaluate locoregional metastasis and/or computed tomography, or positron emission tomography (PET) scans, and brain magnetic resonance imaging (MRI). These will assist with the assessment of tumor extension before surgical excision and sentinel lymph node biopsy. Brain MRI and PET scan are recommended for only very high-risk patients (pT3b and higher)[55]

In patients with positive sentinel lymph node biopsy, the yield of cross-sectional imaging in the detection of clinically occult distant metastasis ranges from 0.5% to 3.7%[56–59] These studies have shown that true positive findings on imaging are most often seen in patients with ulcerated, thick primary melanomas and a large tumor burden noted on the microscopic examination of

their sentinel lymph nodes. The yield of cross-sectional imaging in asymptomatic patients with clinically positive nodes is higher than in patients with positive sentinel lymph nodes[60–62]

While PET scans have shown low yield and poor sensitivity in detecting metastatic disease in patients with clinically localized melanoma, they have been shown to have a role in patients with Stage III disease.[63–65] PET/CT may be able to further characterize lesions that are otherwise indeterminate on CT scan. A systematic review reported a sensitivity ranging from 68% to 87% and specificity ranging from 92% to 98% for Stage III and IV melanoma compared with sensitivity ranging from 0% to 67% and specificity ranging from 77% to 100% for Stage I and II melanoma [66]

## PROGNOSTIC STAGE GROUP

The consequences of melanoma staging to patients are considerable. These include the patients' perception of long-term implications of their health (and quality of life) that is determined by the particular stage that is assigned at the time of diagnosis, and the extent of surgical intervention indicated by staging classification (size of wide local excision, indications for sentinel lymph node biopsy vs therapeutic neck dissection). To that end, recent changes to the AJCC have been shown to have a positive effect on staging and diagnostic concordance compared with the previous edition.[32,47] The AJCC 8th edition provides prognostic stage grouping based on the tumor (T), node (N), and metastasis (M) categories for

---

**Table 6**
**American Joint Committee on Cancer Eighth Edition: M category for Cutaneous Melanoma**

| M Category | M Criteria Anatomic Site | LDH Level |
|---|---|---|
| M0 | No evidence of distant metastasis | Not applicable |
| M1 | Evidence of distant metastasis | See later in discussion |
| M1a M1a(0) M1a(1) | Distant metastasis to skin, soft tissue including muscle, and/ or nonregional lymph node | Not recorded or unspecified Not elevated Elevated |
| M1b M1b(0) M1b(1) | Distant metastasis to lung with or without M1a sites of disease | Not recorded or unspecified Not elevated Elevated |
| M1c M1c(0) M1c(1) | Distant metastasis to non-CNS visceral sites with or without M1a or M1b sites of disease | Not recorded or unspecified Not elevated Elevated |
| M1d M1d(0) M1d(1) | Distant metastasis to CNS with or without M1a, M1b, or M1c sites of disease | Not recorded or unspecified Normal Elevated |

*Data from* Gershenwald JE, Scolyer RA, Hess KR, et al. Melanoma of the skin. In: Amin MB, Edge SB, Greene FL, et al, eds. AJCC Cancer Staging Manual. 7th and 8th eds. New York: Springer International Publishing; 2010 and 2017.

**Table 7**
**American Joint Committee on Cancer Eighth Edition: Clinical Staging cTNM**

| T | N | M | Clinical Stage Group |
|---|---|---|---|
| Tis | N0 | M0 | 0 |
| T1a | N0 | M0 | IA |
| T1b | N0 | M0 | IB |
| T2a | N0 | M0 | IB |
| T2b | N0 | M0 | IIA |
| T3a | N0 | M0 | IIA |
| T3b | N0 | M0 | IIB |
| T4a | N0 | M0 | IIB |
| T4b | N0 | M0 | IIC |
| Any T, Tis | $\geq$N1 | M0 | III |
| Any T | Any N | M1 | IV |

*Data from* Gershenwald JE, Scolyer RA, Hess KR, et al. Melanoma of the skin. In: Amin MB, Edge SB, Greene FL, et al, eds. AJCC Cancer Staging Manual. 7th and 8th eds. New York: Springer International Publishing; 2010 and 2017.

melanoma. Stage groups tend to group patients together based on similar prognosis. Statistically significant differences in outcomes typically separate each group. Patients within each group tend to have similar outcomes. The four-stage groups in the 8th edition are based on multivariable models including T category factors (tumor thickness and ulceration) and N category factors (number of tumor involved nodes, microsatellites, satellites, and in-transit metastases).

## CLINICAL STAGING

As stated earlier, clinical staging occurs following biopsy but before definitive treatment. Clinical staging is based on the initial information or microstaging of the primary tumor (T) and the clinical, radiographic, or biopsy confirmation of regional/nodal (N) or distant metastasis (M). Clinical prognostic stage groups are listed in **Table 7**.

## PATHOLOGIC STAGING (pTNM)

Pathologic staging, (sometimes referred to as the surgical stage) includes information from both the initial biopsy as well as the final specimen (T) following wide local excision. Sentinel lymph

**Table 8**
**American Joint Committee on Cancer Eighth Edition: Pathologic Staging pTNM**

| T | N | M | Pathologic Stage Group |
|---|---|---|---|
| Tis | N0 | M0 | 0 |
| T1a | N0 | M0 | IA |
| T1b | N0 | M0 | IA |
| T2a | N0 | M0 | IB |
| T2b | N0 | M0 | IIA |
| T3a | N0 | M0 | IIA |
| T3b | N0 | M0 | IIB |
| T4a | N0 | M0 | IIB |
| T4b | N0 | M0 | IIC |
| T0 | N1b, N1c | M0 | IIIB |
| T0 | N2b, N2c, N3b, or N3c | M0 | IIIC |
| T1a/b-T2a | N1a or N2a | M0 | IIIA |
| T1a/b-T2a | N1b/c or N2b | M0 | IIIB |
| T2b/T3a | N1a-N2b | M0 | IIIB |
| T1a-T3a | N2c or N3a/b/c | M0 | IIIC |
| T3b/T4a | Any N $\geq$ N1 | M0 | IIIC |
| T4b | N1a-N2c | M0 | IIIC |
| T4b | N3a/b/c | M0 | IIID |
| Any T, Tis | Any N | M1 | IV |

*Data from* Gershenwald JE, Scolyer RA, Hess KR, et al. Melanoma of the skin. In: Amin MB, Edge SB, Greene FL, et al, eds. AJCC Cancer Staging Manual. 7th and 8th eds. New York: Springer International Publishing; 2010 and 2017.

**Table 9**
**Melanoma-specific survival rates**

|  | 5-y Melanoma-Specific Survival Rate (Percentage) | 10-y Melanoma-Specific Survival Rate (Percentage) |
|---|---|---|
| Stage I | 98 | 95 |
| Stage II | 90 | 84 |
| Stage III | 77 | 69 |

*Data from* Gershenwald JE, Scolyer RA. Melanoma Staging: American Joint Committee on Cancer (AJCC) 8th Edition and Beyond. Ann Surg Oncol. 2018 Aug;25(8):2105-2110.

node or therapeutic lymph node dissection will provide histopathologic evidence necessary for N staging. Pathologic prognostic stage groups are listed in **Table 8**.

## MELANOMA-SPECIFIC SURVIVAL RATES

Melanoma-specific survival rates for Stages I-III according to data from AJCC 8th edition[32,67] are shown in **Table 9**. These survival rates have slightly improved from the previous staging system in the 7th edition.[20,32,67] The amount of recent data on survival rates for Stage IV melanoma is limited, and likely underestimated. This is due to previously overall poor survival rates before recent advances in the treatment of metastatic melanoma (including checkpoint inhibitor immunotherapy and molecularly targeted therapy). It is expected that with these new therapies, melanoma-specific survival rates will provide promising data with improved survival rates.

## SUMMARY

Thorough knowledge of the classification and staging of melanoma is paramount to evaluate prognosis, determine the appropriate surgical intervention, and assess eligibility for adjuvant therapy and clinic trials. Of the major melanoma subtypes defined by the WHO, prognostic data are based on the more common subtypes, superficial spreading, and nodular melanoma. Staging of these patients is based on regional nodal status, high-risk pathologic features (tumor thickness and ulceration), and the presence of advanced-stage disease. While other prognostic factors (Clark's level of invasion, mitotic rate) are not incorporated into the current staging system, they still must be recorded for future analysis of prognostic data. The Maxillofacial surgeon must be up to date with the current staging system to provide the most contemporary standard of care for these patients.

## REFERENCES

1. Bray HN, Simpson MC, Zahirsha ZS, et al. Head and Neck Melanoma Incidence Trends in the Pediatric, Adolescent, and Young Adult Population of the United States and Canada, 1995-2014. JAMA Otolaryngology–Head Neck Surg 2019;145(11):1064.
2. Seth R, Messersmith H, Kaur V, et al. Systemic Therapy for Melanoma: ASCO Guideline. J Clin Oncol 2020;38(33). https://doi.org/10.1200/JCO.20.00198.
3. Pulte D, Weberpals J, Jansen L, et al. Changes in population-level survival for advanced solid malignancies with new treatment options in the second decade of the 21st century. Cancer 2019. https://doi.org/10.1002/cncr.32160.
4. McGovern VJ. The classification of melanoma.fusion in dogs. Minn Med 1971;54(6):426–8. Available at: http://www.ncbi.nlm.nih.gov/pubmed/4934440.
5. Clark WH, From L, Bernardino EA, et al. The histogenesis and biologic behavior of primary human malignant melanomas of the skin. Cancer Res 1969;29(3):705–27. Available at: http://www.ncbi.nlm.nih.gov/pubmed/5773814.
6. Elder DE, Bastian BC, Cree IA, et al. The 2018 World Health Organization Classification of Cutaneous, Mucosal, and Uveal Melanoma: Detailed Analysis of 9 Distinct Subtypes Defined by Their Evolutionary Pathway. Arch Pathol Lab Med 2020;144(4):500–22.
7. Massi D, Cree I, Elder DE, et al. WHO classification of skin Tumours.; 2018.
8. Demierre MF, Chung C, Miller DR, et al. Early detection of thick melanomas in the United States: beware of the nodular subtype. Arch Dermatol 2005;141(6). https://doi.org/10.1001/archderm.141.6.745.
9. Coleman WP, Loria PR, Reed RJ, et al. Acral lentiginous melanoma. Arch Dermatol 1980;116(7).
10. Clark WH, Mihm MC. Lentigo maligna and lentigo-maligna melanoma. The Am J Pathol 1969;55(1).
11. Strazzulla LC, Li X, Zhu K, et al. Clinicopathologic, misdiagnosis, and survival differences between clinically amelanotic melanomas and pigmented melanomas. J Am Acad Dermatol 2019;80(5). https://doi.org/10.1016/j.jaad.2019.01.012.

12. Kottschade LA, Grotz TE, Dronca RS, et al. Rare presentations of primary melanoma and special populations: a systematic review. Am J Clin Oncol 2014;37(6). https://doi.org/10.1097/COC.0b013e3182868e82.

13. Lang UE, Yeh I, McCalmont TH. Molecular Melanoma Diagnosis Update: Gene Fusion, Genomic Hybridization, and Massively Parallel Short-Read Sequencing. Clin Lab Med 2017;37(3):473–84.

14. de Unamuno Bustos B, Murria Estal R, Pérez Simó G, et al. Towards Personalized Medicine in Melanoma: Implementation of a Clinical Next-Generation Sequencing Panel. Scientific Rep 2017;7(1):495.

15. Greenhaw BN, Covington KR, Kurley SJ, et al. Molecular risk prediction in cutaneous melanoma: A meta-analysis of the 31-gene expression profile prognostic test in 1,479 patients. J Am Acad Dermatol 2020;83(3):745–53.

16. Grossman D, Okwundu N, Bartlett EK, et al. Prognostic Gene Expression Profiling in Cutaneous Melanoma: Identifying the Knowledge Gaps and Assessing the Clinical Benefit. JAMA Dermatol 2020;156(9):1004–11.

17. Marchetti MA, Coit DG, Dusza SW, et al. Performance of Gene Expression Profile Tests for Prognosis in Patients With Localized Cutaneous Melanoma: A Systematic Review and Meta-analysis. JAMA Dermatol 2020;156(9):953–62.

18. Galan A, Gastman B, Grossmann K, et al. NCCN guidelines version 2.2021 melanoma: cutaneous continue NCCN guidelines Panel Disclosures.; 2021.

19. Siegel RL, Miller KD, Jemal A. Cancer statistics, 2015. CA. A Cancer J Clinicians 2015;65(1). https://doi.org/10.3322/caac.21254.

20. Balch CM, Gershenwald JE, Soong S jaw, et al. Final Version of 2009 AJCC Melanoma Staging and Classification. J Clin Oncol 2009;27(36). https://doi.org/10.1200/JCO.2009.23.4799.

21. Breslow A. Thickness, Cross-Sectional Areas and Depth of Invasion in the Prognosis of Cutaneous Melanoma. Ann Surg 1970;172(5). https://doi.org/10.1097/00000658-197011000-00017.

22. Ge L, Vilain RE, Lo S, et al. Breslow Thickness Measurements of Melanomas Around American Joint Committee on Cancer Staging Cut-Off Points: Imprecision and Terminal Digit Bias Have Important Implications for Staging and Patient Management. Ann Surg Oncol 2016;23(8):2658–63.

23. Gershenwald JE, Scolyer RA, Hess KR, et al. Melanoma staging: Evidence-based changes in the American Joint Committee on Cancer eighth edition cancer staging manual. CA: A Cancer J Clinicians 2017;67(6):472–92.

24. Green AC, Baade P, Coory M, et al. Population-Based 20-Year Survival Among People Diagnosed With Thin Melanomas in Queensland, Australia.

J Clin Oncol 2012;30(13). https://doi.org/10.1200/JCO.2011.38.8561.

25. BALCH CM, MURAD TM, SOONG SJ, et al. A Multifactorial Analysis of Melanoma. Ann Surg 1978;188(6). https://doi.org/10.1097/00000658-197812000-00004.

26. Murali R, Haydu LE, Quinn MJ, et al. Sentinel Lymph Node Biopsy in Patients With Thin Primary Cutaneous Melanoma. Ann Surg 2012;255(1). https://doi.org/10.1097/SLA.0b013e3182306c72.

27. Han D, Zager JS, Shyr Y, et al. Clinicopathologic Predictors of Sentinel Lymph Node Metastasis in Thin Melanoma. J Clin Oncol 2013;31(35). https://doi.org/10.1200/JCO.2013.50.1114.

28. Cordeiro E, Gervais MK, Shah PS, et al. Sentinel Lymph Node Biopsy in Thin Cutaneous Melanoma: A Systematic Review and Meta-Analysis. Ann Surg Oncol 2016;23(13). https://doi.org/10.1245/s10434-016-5137-z.

29. Andtbacka RHI, Gershenwald JE. Role of Sentinel Lymph Node Biopsy in Patients with Thin Melanoma. J Natl Compr Cancer Netw 2009;7(3). https://doi.org/10.6004/jnccn.2009.0023.

30. Portelli F, Galli F, Cattaneo L, et al. The prognostic impact of the extent of ulceration in patients with clinical stage I– <scp>II</scp> melanoma: a multi-centre study of the Italian Melanoma Intergroup ( <scp>IMI</scp> ). Br J Dermatol 2021;(2):184. https://doi.org/10.1111/bjd.19120.

31. Balch CM, Wilkerson JA, Murad TM, et al. The prognostic significance of ulceration of cutaneous melanoma. Cancer 1980;45(12). https://doi.org/10.1002/1097-0142(19800615)45:12<3012::AID-CNCR2820451223>3.0.

32. Gershenwald JE, Scolyer RA, Hess KR, et al. Melanoma of the Skin. In: AJCC Cancer staging manual. Springer International Publishing; 2017. https://doi.org/10.1007/978-3-319-40618-3_47.

33. Scolyer RA, Rawson Rv, Gershenwald JE, et al. Melanoma pathology reporting and staging. Mod Pathol 2020;33(S1). https://doi.org/10.1038/s41379-019-0402-x.

34. 't Hout FEM, Haydu LE, Murali R, et al. Prognostic Importance of the Extent of Ulceration in Patients With Clinically Localized Cutaneous Melanoma. Ann Surg 2012;255(6). https://doi.org/10.1097/SLA.0b013e31824c4b0b.

35. Mandalà M, Galli F, Cattaneo L, et al. Mitotic rate correlates with sentinel lymph node status and outcome in cutaneous melanoma greater than 1 millimeter in thickness: A multi-institutional study of 1524 cases. J Am Acad Dermatol 2017;76(2). https://doi.org/10.1016/j.jaad.2016.08.066.

36. Thompson JF, Soong SJ, Balch CM, et al. Prognostic Significance of Mitotic Rate in Localized Primary Cutaneous Melanoma: An Analysis of Patients in the Multi-Institutional American Joint Committee on

Cancer Melanoma Staging Database. J Clin Oncol 2011;29(16). https://doi.org/10.1200/JCO.2010.31.5812.

37. Tejera-Vaquerizo A, Ribero S, Puig S, et al. Survival analysis and sentinel lymph node status in thin cutaneous melanoma: A multicenter observational study. Cancer Med 2019;8(9). https://doi.org/10.1002/cam4.2358.

38. Wong SL, Balch CM, Hurley P, et al. Sentinel Lymph Node Biopsy for Melanoma: American Society of Clinical Oncology and Society of Surgical Oncology Joint Clinical Practice Guideline. J Clin Oncol 2012; 30(23). https://doi.org/10.1200/JCO.2011.40.3519.

39. de Rosa N, Lyman GH, Silbermins D, et al. Sentinel Node Biopsy for Head and Neck Melanoma. Otolaryngology–Head Neck Surg 2011;145(3). https://doi.org/10.1177/0194599811408554.

40. Wong SL, Faries MB, Kennedy EB, et al. Sentinel Lymph Node Biopsy and Management of Regional Lymph Nodes in Melanoma: American Society of Clinical Oncology and Society of Surgical Oncology Clinical Practice Guideline Update. J Clin Oncol 2018;36(4). https://doi.org/10.1200/JCO.2017.75.7724.

41. Lee CC, Faries MB, Wanek LA, et al. Improved Survival After Lymphadenectomy for Nodal Metastasis From an Unknown Primary Melanoma. J Clin Oncol 2008;26(4). https://doi.org/10.1200/JCO.2007.14.0285.

42. van der Ploeg APT, Haydu LE, Spillane AJ, et al. Melanoma Patients with an Unknown Primary Tumor Site Have a Better Outcome than Those with a Known Primary Following Therapeutic Lymph Node Dissection for Macroscopic (Clinically Palpable) Nodal Disease. Ann Surg Oncol 2014;21(9). https://doi.org/10.1245/s10434-014-3679-5.

43. Schröer-Günther MA, Wolff RF, Westwood ME, et al. F-18-fluoro-2-deoxyglucose positron emission tomography (PET) and PET/computed tomography imaging in primary staging of patients with malignant melanoma: a systematic review. Syst Rev 2012;1(1). https://doi.org/10.1186/2046-4053-1-62.

44. Rao UNM, Ibrahim J, Flaherty LE, et al. Implications of Microscopic Satellites of the Primary and Extracapsular Lymph Node Spread in Patients With High-Risk Melanoma: Pathologic Corollary of Eastern Cooperative Oncology Group Trial E1690. J Clin Oncol 2002; 20(8). https://doi.org/10.1200/JCO.2002.08.024.

45. Read RL, Haydu L, Saw RPM, et al. In-transit Melanoma Metastases: Incidence, Prognosis, and the Role of Lymphadenectomy. Ann Surg Oncol 2015; 22(2). https://doi.org/10.1245/s10434-014-4100-0.

46. Frishberg DP, Balch C, Balzer BL, et al. Protocol for the Examination of Specimens From Patients With Melanoma of the Skin. Arch Pathol Lab Med 2009; 133(10). https://doi.org/10.5858/133.10.1560.

47. Balch CM, Gershenwald JE, Soong SJ, et al. Final version of 2009 AJCC melanoma staging and classification. J Clin Oncol 2009;27(36):6199–206. https://doi.org/10.1200/JCO.2009.23.4799.

48. Sirott MN, Bajorin DF, Wong GY, et al. Prognostic factors in patients with metastatic malignant melanoma. A Multivariate Analysis Cancer 1993;72(10). https://doi.org/10.1002/1097-0142(19931115)72:10<3091::aid-cncr2820721034>3.0.co;2-v.

49. Manola J, Atkins M, Ibrahim J, et al. Prognostic Factors in Metastatic Melanoma: A Pooled Analysis of Eastern Cooperative Oncology Group Trials. J Clin Oncol 2000;18(22). https://doi.org/10.1200/JCO.2000.18.22.3782.

50. Keilholz U, Martus P, Punt CJA, et al. Prognostic factors for survival and factors associated with long-term remission in patients with advanced melanoma receiving cytokine-based treatments. Eur J Cancer 2002;38(11). https://doi.org/10.1016/S0959-8049(02)00123-5.

51. Bedikian AY, Johnson MM, Warneke CL, et al. Prognostic Factors That Determine the Long-Term Survival of Patients with Unresectable Metastatic Melanoma. Cancer Invest 2008;26(6). https://doi.org/10.1080/07357900802027073.

52. Larkin J, Chiarion-Sileni V, Gonzalez R, et al. Five-Year Survival with Combined Nivolumab and Ipilimumab in Advanced Melanoma. N Engl J Med 2019; 381(16). https://doi.org/10.1056/NEJMoa1910836.

53. Kelderman S, Heemskerk B, van Tinteren H, et al. Lactate dehydrogenase as a selection criterion for ipilimumab treatment in metastatic melanoma. Cancer Immunol Immunother 2014. https://doi.org/10.1007/s00262-014-1528-9.

54. Diem S, Kasenda B, Spain L, et al. Serum lactate dehydrogenase as an early marker for outcome in patients treated with anti-PD-1 therapy in metastatic melanoma. Br J Cancer 2016;114(3):256–61.

55. Michielin O, van Akkooi ACJ, Ascierto PA, et al. Cutaneous melanoma: ESMO Clinical Practice Guidelines for diagnosis, treatment and follow-up †. Ann Oncol 2019. https://doi.org/10.1093/annonc/mdz411.

56. Buzaid AC, Tinoco L, Ross MI, et al. Role of computed tomography in the staging of patients with local-regional metastases of melanoma. J Clin Oncol 1995;13(8). https://doi.org/10.1200/JCO.1995.13.8.2104.

57. Johnson TM, Fader DJ, Chang AE, et al. Computed tomography in staging of patients with melanoma metastatic to the regional nodes. Ann Surg Oncol 1997;4(5). https://doi.org/10.1007/BF02305552.

58. Kuvshinoff BW, Kurtz C, Coit DG. Computed tomography in evaluation of patients with stage III melanoma. Ann Surg Oncol 1997;4(3). https://doi.org/10.1007/BF02306618.

59. Pandalai PK, Dominguez FJ, Michaelson J, et al. Clinical Value of Radiographic Staging in Patients Diagnosed With AJCC Stage III Melanoma. Ann

Surg Oncol 2011;18(2). https://doi.org/10.1245/s10434-010-1272-0.

60. Aloia TA, Gershenwald JE, Andtbacka RH, et al. Utility of Computed Tomography and Magnetic Resonance Imaging Staging Before Completion Lymphadenectomy in Patients With Sentinel Lymph Node–Positive Melanoma. J Clin Oncol 2006; 24(18). https://doi.org/10.1200/JCO.2006.05.6176.

61. Gold JS, Jaques DP, Busam KJ, et al. Yield and Predictors of Radiologic Studies for Identifying Distant Metastases in Melanoma Patients with a Positive Sentinel Lymph Node Biopsy. Ann Surg Oncol 2007; 14(7). https://doi.org/10.1245/s10434-007-9399-3.

62. Miranda EP. Routine Imaging of Asymptomatic Melanoma Patients With Metastasis to Sentinel Lymph Nodes Rarely Identifies Systemic Disease. Arch Surg 2004;139(8). https://doi.org/10.1001/archsurg.139.8.831.

63. Maubec E, Lumbroso J, Masson F, et al. F-18 fluorodeoxy-D-glucose positron emission tomography scan in the initial evaluation of patients with a primary melanoma thicker than 4mm. Melanoma Res 2007;17(3). https://doi.org/10.1097/CMR.0b013e32815c10b0.

64. Wagner JD, Schauwecker D, Davidson D, et al. Inefficacy of F-18 fluorodeoxy-D-glucose-positron emission tomography scans for initial evaluation in early-stage cutaneous melanoma. Cancer 2005;104(3). https://doi.org/10.1002/cncr.21189.

65. Bikhchandani J, Wood J, Richards AT, et al. No benefit in staging fluorodeoxyglucose-positron emission tomography in clinically node-negative head and neck cutaneous melanoma. Head & Neck 2013. https://doi.org/10.1002/hed.23456.

66. Clark PB. Futility of Fluorodeoxyglucose F 18 Positron Emission Tomography in Initial Evaluation of Patients With T2 to T4 Melanoma. Arch Surg 2006; 141(3). https://doi.org/10.1001/archsurg.141.3.284.

67. Gershenwald JE, Scolyer RA. Melanoma Staging: American Joint Committee on Cancer (AJCC) 8th Edition and Beyond. Ann Surg Oncol. 25. 2017. doi:10.1245/s10434-018-6513-7.

# Imaging and Laboratory Workup for Melanoma

Arshad Kaleem, DMD, MD[a], Neel Patel, DMD, MD[a],*,
Srinivasa Rama Chandra, BDS, MD, FDSRCS(Eng), FIBCSOMS(Onc-Recon)[b],
R.L. Vijayaraghavan, MD, DNB[c]

## KEYWORDS

- Melanoma • Metastasis • CT • MRI • PET • Ultrasound • LDH • S100B

## KEY POINTS

- Imaging and laboratory work have no role in the workup of early-stage melanoma nor in routine surveillance.
- Computed tomography (CT) and MRI play roles in melanoma workup; however, they have site-specific limitations.
- Fused PET/CT and PET/MRI improve the diagnostic accuracy compared with PET alone in the detection of metastatic disease.
- Single-photon emission tomography/CT improves the nodal detection rates compared with planar lymphoscintigraphy in sentinel lymph node workup.
- Lactate dehydrogenase represents a reliable serum biomarker in late-stage melanoma. S100B continues to be studied and may represent a helpful marker in intermediate to late-stage disease.

## INTRODUCTION

Skin cancer represents by far the most common cancer in the world, and among those, melanoma represents about 1% of all skin cancers. However, melanoma accounts for most deaths related to skin cancer.[1] Approximately 80% to 85% of patients diagnosed with melanoma without evidence of metastasis survive at least 5 years, indicating that about 15% to 20% of patients without clinical signs of metastasis die from progression of disease and occult metastasis within 5 years, thus representing a significant rate of mortality from this type of cancer. Therefore, a thorough and comprehensive workup is always warranted to rule out metastatic disease.[2] Patients with early-stage melanoma have favorable outcomes following complete surgical resection. However, about 50% to 80% of patients with locoregional disease and almost all patients with distant metastasis experience recurrence after primary treatment.[3] Hence, management of patients with advanced metastatic disease has been a challenge. The most common sites of metastasis in decreasing frequency are skin, lymph nodes, lungs, liver, brain, bone, and gastrointestinal tract.[4] Physical examination remains the mainstay of the initial evaluation, particularly in localized disease, and in evaluation of local and regional lymph nodes, although it is relatively insensitive and has limited use for detection of metastasis in visceral sites. Unlike squamous cell carcinoma of the head and neck where imaging is used for both assessment of local disease and regional involvement, imaging and laboratory studies in melanoma are used primarily to assist in detection of locoregional and distant metastatic disease once the diagnosis of melanoma has been made. This

[a] DeWitt Daughtry Family Department of Surgery, Division of Oral and Maxillofacial Surgery, Section of Head and Neck Surgical Oncology & Microvascular Reconstructive Surgery, University of Miami Miller School of Medicine, Jackson Health System, Deering Medical Plaza, 9380 Southwest 150th Street #170, Miami, FL 33176, USA; [b] Department of Oral and Maxillofacial Surgery, Oregon Health and Sciences University, 2730 S Moody Avenue, Portland, OR 97201, USA; [c] Department of Molecular Imaging and Radionuclide Therapy, Nanjappa Life Care Super-specialty Hospital, 5619 Sagar Road, Gadikoppa, Shivamogga, Karnataka 577205, India
* Corresponding author.

Oral Maxillofacial Surg Clin N Am 34 (2022) 235–250
https://doi.org/10.1016/j.coms.2021.11.004
1042-3699/22/© 2021 Elsevier Inc. All rights reserved.

article focuses on the advanced imaging techniques and laboratory evaluations that can be used in the workup and staging of melanoma of the head and neck.

## IMAGING

The use of imaging studies in the diagnostic workup of both cutaneous and mucosal melanoma of the head and neck is crucial to obtain the appropriate staging. Imaging can be used to assess the extent of disease at the initial presentation, detect and evaluate recurrence, and monitor disease progression, regression, and response to treatment. In routine workup, a variety of imaging modalities can be used, such as plain films, computed tomography (CT), ultrasound (US), fluorodeoxyglucose (FDG) -PET, MRI, or a combination of these.

Historically, plain chest radiographs have been used to evaluate potential involvement of the lungs, as this is the most common visceral site of metastasis, and because of the ease of obtaining this study.[5] A retrospective study conducted by Terhune and colleagues[6] showed chest radiographs are not beneficial, especially in stage I and II melanoma, and in asymptomatic patients. Chest radiographs yield true positive rates of about 0.1% and, in fact, have in other studies yielded false positive and inconclusive rates as high as 8% to 15%.[7] When melanoma spreads to the lungs, it often will appear as multiple subcentimeter foci,[8,9] and as such, because the resolution of plain films is limited to lesions that measure at least 1 cm or greater,[10] they do not possess the level of sensitivity necessary to detect small metastatic foci. As such, the Clinical Practice Guidelines in Melanoma released by the National Comprehensive Cancer Network no longer state the recommendation of plain chest films in a standard head and neck melanoma workup. In patients with pulmonary symptoms or higher-stage disease, however, plain chest films may play a role in the initial workup.

CT of the chest, on the other hand, has shown that it is superior to plain chest films in detection of pulmonary metastasis, in particular in high-risk individuals, and has been shown to be about 20% higher than plain films.[11] A study by Silverman and colleagues[12] looked at 70 symptomatic patients with Clark level III, IV, and V melanoma using CT imaging, and metastatic disease was detected in lymph nodes in 24%, 33%, and 75% of patients with Clark level III, IV, and V melanoma, respectively, as well as hepatic and splenic metastasis in 25% of patients with Clark level V disease. However, the routine use of CT scanning in low-risk individuals, such as those with stage I and II disease, has not been recommended because of low detection rates and high rate of false positives, which have been shown to be up to 17%.[13] In a study by Buzaid in 1995,[14] 89 symptomatic patients with clinical evidence of lymphatic metastasis all had normal chest films, and chest CT images revealed a true positive rate of 6.7% and a false positive rate of 22%, with only detection of 1 patient (1.1%) via CT scan where the plain film was negative. Abdominal and pelvic CTs in this study revealed only 5.6% true positives. If CT scans are used, an image taken after intravenous contrast has been administered increases the sensitivity significantly, as metastatic melanoma is hypervascular, and thus, lesions appear hyperdense on early-phase contrast-enhanced CT.[15] Multiple-phase imaging consists of several sets of CT images obtained at different times following contrast injection to increase the detection of metastatic melanoma, ideally with 2 image sets, 1 set before contrast injection and the second set during the portal venous phase (60 seconds following the start of contrast injection).[16] Despite this, the use of CT scans of the head, neck, chest, abdomen, and pelvis in detection of metastatic melanoma has demonstrated poorly reliable results and thus is not routinely recommended in both localized lesions and tumors with evidence of locoregional lymphatic spread.[17]

The use of MRI in the workup of patients with melanoma has been well established, in particular, the use of whole-body MRI techniques with diffusion-weighted imaging (DWI). The lack of ionizing radiation and whole-body coverage make it an attractive option in evaluation of metastatic disease. DWI reflects the movement of water molecules in the tissues owing to their random thermal motion, and restriction of water diffusion is inversely associated with the integrity of cell membranes and tissue cellularity.[18] This provides functional information and is used for the detection of pathologic condition, in particular, processes such as acute cerebral infarction and malignant tumors.[19] The imaging characteristics of metastatic melanoma are distinct; with the presence of melanin and propensity for hemorrhage, they result in T1-weighted signal hyperintensity and T2-weighted signal intensity loss.[20] In a comparison of whole-body MRI with DWI and CT scanning in detection of metastatic melanoma, Mosav and colleagues[21] found that CT scans performed better than MRI scans in the detection of thoracic metastasis (lungs, mediastinal lymph nodes), likely because of the cardiac and respiratory motion artifact (Fig. 1). However, in the detection of abdominal and bone metastasis, MRI performed considerably better than CT. Cerebral metastatic involvement in cases of advanced melanoma carries with it a significantly higher mortality, with patients that have melanoma brain metastases having a median overall survival of about 4 to 6 months, or less than 2 months if leptomeningeal involvement is present[22]; thus, accurate detection of brain involvement is crucial. Melanoma represents the third most common cause of brain masses with an unknown primary[23] and should always be considered in these cases. Recommendations currently for stage IIIc and higher melanomas involve imaging of the brain in the form of an MRI with and without gadolinium contrast at the outset of diagnosis, because of the higher risk of brain involvement, with MRI being the preferred method for evaluation of the brain.[24] Tyler and colleagues[25] demonstrated that the incidence of brain metastasis at the time of diagnosis is very low at about 0.2% (46 out of 19,066 patients), although this number has been shown in the literature to be as high as 5%,[26] and the risk of brain involvement increases as time goes on and thus must be assessed, especially in high-risk patients.

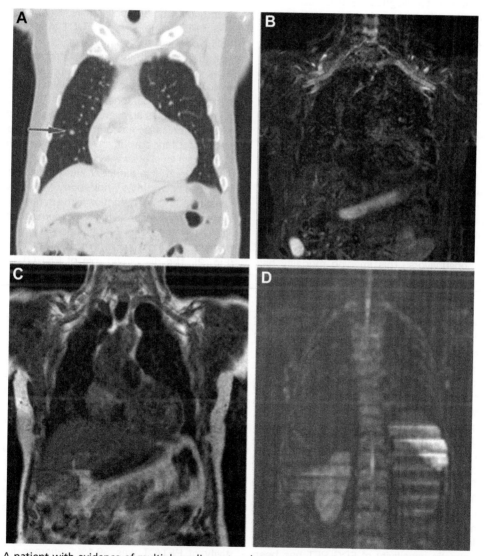

**Fig. 1.** A patient with evidence of multiple malignant melanoma metastases. CT image (A) shows lesion in the right lung measuring 7 mm in diameter. The lesion was not detectable on short tau inversion recovery and T1-weighted imaging (B, C), nor could it be detected on coronal maximum intensity projection DWI image (D). From Mosavi F, Ullenhag G, Ahlström H. Whole-body MRI including diffusion-weighted imaging compared to CT for staging of malignant melanoma. Ups J Med Sci. 2013 May;118(2):91-7.)

Vital cell signaling pathways can explain the aggressive nature of the tumor biology in melanoma. About 90% of melanomas involves activating oncogene mutations in the MAPK pathway. The MAPK pathway plays a significant role in coordinating the differentiation and proliferation of melanocytes. About 50% of patients with melanoma demonstrates mutations in BRAF-V600; about 20% shows NRAS mutation; 14% shows NF1 gene mutation, and 3% to 5% of patients harbor activating KIT mutation.[27–29] These mutations lead to overexpression of GLUT1 receptors, which forms the basis of imaging with FDG-PET. This imaging modality has been shown to have a role in initial diagnosis and workup in the assessment and staging of melanoma, demonstrating the increased tissue metabolism and uptake of the 18F-FDG radiotracer in metastatic lesions. Metabolic parameters in FDG-PET imaging, such as maximum standardized uptake value (SUVmax), metabolic tumor volume (MTV), and total lesion glycolysis (TLG), are used as prognosticators. SUVmax is a semiquantitative parameter that represents pixels with the highest glucose uptake. MTV is a distal volumetric assessment of FDG uptake within the lesion, whereas TLG is obtained by multiplying the mean SUV across the lesion with MTV. A retrospective review conducted by Son and colleagues[30] showed that in 41 biopsy-proven cases of cutaneous melanoma, the SUVmax and TLG in staging FDG-PET were higher in patients who presented with recurrence and in nonsurvivors. This imaging modality has been shown to be particularly useful in more advanced stage III and higher melanomas, where its role has been demonstrated to influence the management of 22% to 49% of stage III and IV cases.[31] In contrast, the use of FDG-PET in staging of early cases of melanoma has not been recommended because of the lack of sensitivity in detection of lesions.[32] Wagner and colleagues[33] conducted a prospective study involving 70 patients with melanoma greater than 1 mm thickness and 4 patients with locally recurrent melanoma, and FDG-PET and sentinel lymph node biopsy (SLNB) were performed. PET/CT demonstrated a specificity of 100%; however, it had poor sensitivity. They also concluded that FDG-PET could not reliably detect metastasis in lymph nodes smaller than 80 mm$^3$. PET/CT may not be useful in the initial staging of skin melanoma without clinical evidence of local or distant metastasis.[34–38] The diagnostic sensitivity of FDG-PET has been shown to be approximately 90% for metastatic lesions that are greater than 78 mm$^3$ in volume (>5.3 mm in diameter),[39,40] and thus, PET alone is unable to accurately detect micrometastasis. A study conducted by McIvor et al[41] did however demonstrate a 17% detection rate of occult metastasis by PET alone in a group of 322 patients with stage I or II disease, with 43% of those having distant metastasis with or without nodal disease. Thus, the use of PET scanning alone has shown limited value in detection of metastatic disease in melanoma, in particular, in its early stages. The fusion of PET imaging with other modalities, such as CT or MRI, has demonstrated an improved performance in detection of distant disease in the patient with melanoma, and continues to show promise, as it combines anatomic as well as physiologic information of the tissues that increases the effectiveness in detecting metastatic disease.[42] In a study by Krug and colleagues,[43] comparing the use of PET alone versus PET/CT in stage III and higher disease, the combination of PET/CT performed better with increased detection of metastatic disease, with sensitivity and specificity of up to 83% and 85%, respectively. Furthermore, it has also been demonstrated that PET/CT imaging demonstrates an overall improved detection of metastatic disease as compared with whole-body MRI, except for brain involvement, where MRI has the highest level of sensitivity in detection of suspicious lesions.[44] In the latter study, a site-specific analysis showed that whole-body MRI was more sensitive for tumor detection in the central nervous system, liver, as well as the bone marrow, whereas PET/CT was superior for detection of lymph node metastases and involvement of all other organs (**Fig. 2**). The diagnostic role of PET/CT has not been substantially evaluated in early stages of malignant melanoma (stage I and II), and considering the relatively high rate of PET/CT false positives and low rate of nodal disease (less than 15%) as well as distant metastasis (less than 5%) at the time of primary diagnosis in these cases,[45,46] PET/CT does not yet represent a standard of care in these cases, as SLNB is the preferred method of initial staging in these early cases.[47] Nevertheless, some studies have demonstrated a high diagnostic accuracy for PET/CT in the detection of metastasis in patients with high-risk melanoma with stage I or II disease, with sensitivities of 91% and 98%.[48,49] The use of PET/MRI has also gained favor in some institutions, given its improved soft tissue imaging capability as compared with CT. In a direct comparison of PET/CT and PET/MRI done in patients with melanoma by Berzaczy and colleagues,[50] the sensitivity of PET/CT was 89.1%, whereas for PET/MRI was 92.7% with specificities equal at 100% for both; however, these results were not found to be statistically significant. Site-specific analysis revealed that although PET/MRI may be more

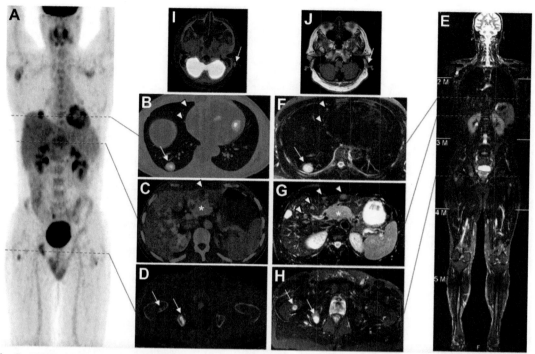

**Fig. 2.** PET/CT (*A–D*) and whole-body MRI (*E–H*) of patient with metastatic malignant melanoma. CT and MRI detected more lung metastasis than PET/CT (*B* and *F, arrows*), and MRI found more liver lesions than PET/CT (*C* and *G, arrows*). Bone metastasis was equally detected (*D* and *H, arrows*). Nodal metastasis behind the left ear (*I* and *J, arrows*) was detected solely by PET/CT. (*From* Pfannenberg C, Aschoff P, Schanz S, Eschmann SM, Plathow C, Eigentler TK, Garbe C, Brechtel K, Vonthein R, Bares R, Claussen CD, Schlemmer HP. Prospective comparison of 18F-fluorodeoxyglucose positron emission tomography/computed tomography and whole-body magnetic resonance imaging in staging of advanced malignant melanoma. Eur J Cancer. 2007 Feb;43(3):557-64; with permission.)

sensitive for melanoma metastasis in some tissues, such as bone, brain, and liver, it does not do as well as PET/CT for evaluation of lung and lymph node metastases (**Fig. 3**).[51] Given this, it may be extrapolated that PET/MRI may be more useful in higher-stage (stage III or above) melanoma, because it appears to be more sensitive in sites where detection of tumor may result in changes in therapeutic modalities (ie, radiation therapy for brain and bone metastasis). Despite the promising results seen with fused imaging modalities, they have been shown to continually be inferior to SLNB and thus cannot replace the latter as the preferred method of diagnosis and staging.[52]

The most important prognostic factor in early-stage melanoma is metastasis to local and regional lymph nodes, and thus, identification of involved nodes is crucial in the workup process.[53] Nuclear imaging finds utility in staging and prognostication, evaluation of recurrence, and response assessment to personalized, targeted therapy. The use of SLNB has been well established in the literature as a reliable method to determine lymphatic spread and is recommended to be used starting in stage IB tumors.[54,55] This procedure was first introduced in 1953 and then was made popular in a large international study entitled the Multicenter Selective Lymphadenectomy Trial, which notably showed that patients with positive sentinel nodes (SNs) who proceeded to have completion lymph node dissection had double the disease-specific survival and triple the disease-free survival.[56] Lymphoscintigraphy represents an inexpensive, relatively noninvasive, and sensitive imaging technique (approximately 95%)[57] for identification of nodal drainage patterns and guidance for SLNB procedures, delivering a low dose of radiation to the patient in the process. It is performed in patients with intermediate-risk primary lesions (1.0–4.0 mm lesion thickness) and clinically nonpalpable regional lymph nodes (cN0 disease) and helps in localization and biopsy of sentinel lymph nodes (SLN) that drain the primary tumor. It is well known that metastasis to locoregional lymph nodes is an essential predictor of recurrence in melanoma,[36] and as such, biopsy-proven metastasis to an SLN would prompt

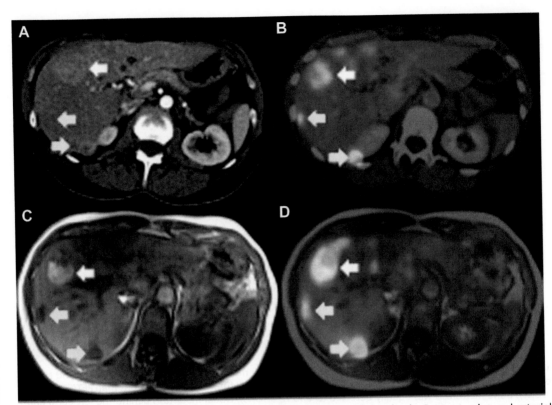

**Fig. 3.** Patient after surgical resection of primary nodular melanoma of the cheek. Contrast-enhanced arterial phase CT (*A*) and corresponding fused PET/CT images (*B*); at least 5 hepatic lesions (*white and yellow arrows*) are seen. PET/MRI images (*C*) also reveal multiple partly hyperintense lesions owing to melanin contact or intra-lesional hemorrhage (*white arrow*), with a pathologic focal tracer uptake on the PET component of the fused PET/MRI image (*D*). (*From* Berzaczy D, Fueger B, Hoeller C, Haug AR, Staudenherz A, Berzaczy G, Weber M, Mayerhoe-fer ME. Whole-Body [18F]FDG-PET/MRI vs. [18F]FDG-PET/CT in Malignant Melanoma. Mol Imaging Biol. 2020 Jun;22(3):739-744; with permission.)

regional lymph node dissection. If SLNB does not show metastasis on histopathological examination, such cases can be spared lymph node dissection. The SLN lymphoscintigraphy proced-ure (**Box 1**) and biopsy remain the standard for staging locoregional lymph nodal involvement. This procedure can be performed either in a -one or a 2-day technique, with the 1-day method requiring a single injection of radionuclide for both diagnostic lymphoscintigraphy and surgery, whereas the 2-day technique requires 2 injections separated by 24 hours, with surgery performed with a gamma probe to aid in localization of nodes with radiotracer. In addition, a blue dye may be injected into the lesion at the time of surgery, and lymphatic drainage patterns are observed to aid in identification of nodal basins and have been shown to be a complementary procedure to lymphoscintigraphy, with an 80% sensitivity.[58] In the head and neck, however, reliable and accu-rate observation of lymphatic spread is much more difficult because of the complex anatomy and

variability of lymphatics, which can result in higher rates of false negative results (reported up to 44%)[59] in comparison with tumors in other sites in the body.[60–62] Introduction of the use of single-photon emission tomography/computed tomography (SPECT/CT) in combination with lym-phoscintigraphy aids in better nodal localization by demonstrating anatomic tomographic slices of radiotracer distribution in the tissues, increasing the likelihood of SLN detection and removal of any positive nodes.[63] In a recent study by Kwak and colleagues,[64] the "hottest" node seen on SPECT/CT was also the "hottest" node intraoper-atively using the gamma probe in 85% of patients. Moreover, the use of this imaging technique in combination with lymphoscintigraphy has shown a significant impact on surgical approach, particu-larly in head and neck melanoma, as studies have shown a change of 41.6% and 49.38% in surgical management based on findings of SPECT/CT-enhanced SLNB as opposed to the use of lympho-scintigraphy alone.[65,66] Some of the advantages of

---

**Box 1**
**Outline of lymphoscintigraphy procedure**

Lymphoscintigraphy

Radiopharmaceutical:

- *$^{99m}$Tc-sulfur colloid* is the most commonly used radiopharmaceutical.
- It can be filtered with a 100-nm to 200-nm membrane filter to obtain particles of uniform size.
- Other radiopharmaceuticals used are $^{99m}$Tc-dextran (mean particle size 2–3 nm), $^{99m}$Tc-DTPA mannosyl dextran (mean particle size 6–8 nm), $^{99m}$Tc-labeled human serum albumin colloid, $^{99m}$Tc-human serum albumin (mean particle size 2–3 nm).

Preparation of $^{99m}$Tc-sulphur colloid:

The preparation kit comprises 3 different components:

- *Component A*: 0.5 mL of 0.3 N HCl (hydrochloric acid)
- *Component B*: 1 mL of solution with 10% sodium thiosulphate and 3.5% gelatin
- *Component C*: 1 mL of 0.08 M phosphate buffer at pH 7.4 with 136 mg of $Na_2HPO_4$ and 12 mg of $NaH_2PO_4$
- *Components A and C* are stored at room temperature, and *component B* has to be refrigerated at 2°C-8°C

Radiolabeling[70–72]:

- A maximum of 100 μCi (3.7 MBq) of $^{99m}$Tco$_4^-$ in 3-mL solution is added to component A. This cocktail forms the *reaction vial.*
- 0.5 mL of component B is transferred to the reaction vial. It is mixed well and placed in a boiling water bath for 3 to 5 minutes.
- The vial is allowed to cool to room temperature (5 minutes).
- 0.5 mL of component C is then transferred into the reaction vial and mixed well.
- $^{99m}$Tc-sulfur colloid will be ready for use after 5 minutes.

Labeling features:

- A 99mTc-sulphur colloid in colloidal suspension
- pH 4 to 7
- Radiochemical purity: greater than 95%
- Free pertechnetate ($^{99m}$Tco$_4^-$): less than 5%

Quality control procedure:

- Radiochemical purity is assessed by ascending chromatography using instant thin-layer chromatography or Whatman no. 1 paper.
- RF (relative front) values in acetone or saline for $^{99m}$Tc-sulfur colloid is 0.0–0.1 and for $^{99m}$Tco$_4$ is 0.9–1.0.

Dosimetry:

- Current dosimetric data are obtained from SLN lymphoscintigraphy procedures in breast cancer.[73,74]
- Radiation dose to the patient depends on (a) amount of injected dose; (b) time to surgery.
- The recommended dose for injection: ranges from 15-Mbq (single-day procedure) to 120-MBq (2-day procedure) in a total volume of 0.4 to 1.0 mL. The intention is to achieve at least activity of 10 MBq at the time of surgery.
- Most centers perform SLNB within 24 hours of lymphoscintigraphy.
- The safety of SLNB is confirmed by studies from Memorial Sloan Kettering Cancer Center. The effective dose from the procedure is calculated to be around 0.2 mSv.[75]

Procedure:

- Patients should be informed about the procedure, discomfort involved, and potential risk of bleeding. Written informed consent must be obtained before the procedure.

- *Injection*: Tuberculin syringe with 25- or 27-gauge needle and minimal dead space are recommended (**Fig. 4**).
- *Activity for injection*: Varies from 15 to 120 MBq between studies.
- *Site*: Tracer should be injected at about 0.1 to 0.5 cm from the tumor margin.
- Aliquots vary according to the size and location of the tumor.
- Tumors in the floor of the mouth require 4 separate submucosal injections around the lesion.
- For tumors in other head and neck noncutaneous sites like tongue, a tracer should be injected according to the depth of the lesion too.
- The first-echelon and second-echelon lymph nodes should separately be marked on the skin using indelible markers of different colors, guided by a gamma camera and a handheld gamma probe or a radioactive point source (**Fig. 5**).
- *Dynamic and static images should be taken, and topographic localization using $^{57}$Co flood source for simultaneous emission and transmission imaging and SPECT/CT should be performed* (**Figs. 6–9**).
- The patient should be asked to rinse the oral cavity after injection to prevent the pooling of the tracer.

SPECT/CT include the following: (a) identification of missed SLN and exclusion of ambiguous SLN; (b) compared with planar imaging, SPECT/CT identifies at least 1 additional lymph node; (c) better anatomic localization in 30% to 47% cases; (d) it can identify SLN located close to the primary tumor, which is commonly missed by the intraoperative gamma probe; (e) high-quality CT helps identify subcentimeter SLN and hence improved intraoperative SLN localization. The benefits of SPECT/CT have not been universally accepted; however, both planar and SPECT/CT images have been shown to demonstrate good interobserver and intraobserver agreement for evaluation of SLN,[67] with kappa values ranging from 0.68 to 0.89. This procedure is not without its risks of adverse and/or allergic reactions, as such reactions to human serum albumin colloid have been

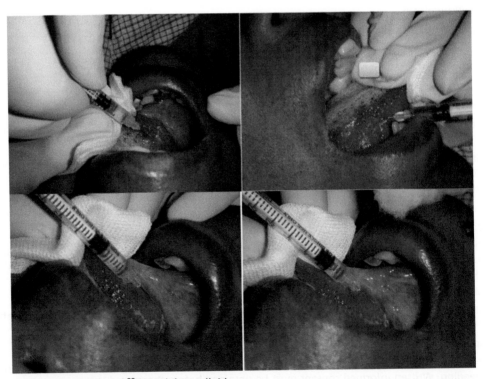

**Fig. 4.** Peritumoral injection of $^{99m}$Tc-sulphur colloid.

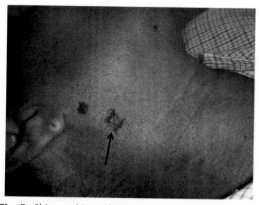

**Fig. 5.** Skin marking of SLN.

reported in the literature.[68,69] Another group wherein caution must be taken is in pregnant and lactating women, with associated potential risks to the child. Fetal-absorbed dose from a tracer activity of 18.5 MBq has been calculated to be 0.013 mSv, with congenital malformations primarily observed at exposures greater than 200 mSV. Given this, SLNB is not contraindicated during pregnancy; however, it is preferable to perform a single-day procedure with a lower injected dose. In lactating women, it is advised that they stop breastfeeding for 24 hours following SLNB procedures.

The use of US in patients with melanoma has been shown to have multiple applications, in assessment of the primary tumor itself as well as in detection of regional metastasis. It is well known that the thickness of melanoma is a major prognostic factor and also determines the margins of surgical excision. High-resolution US imaging has been used to accurately measure tumor thickness and has shown promising results. A systematic review by Machet and colleagues[76] that included 14 studies compared both US and

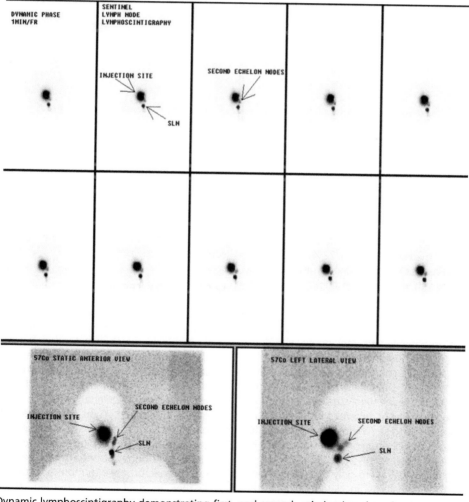

**Fig. 6.** Dynamic lymphoscintigraphy demonstrating first- and second- echelon lymph nodes.

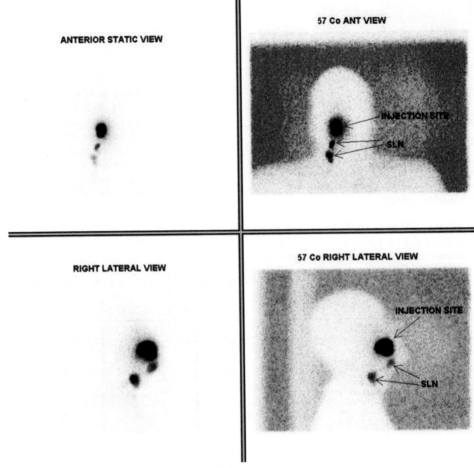

**Fig. 7.** Topographic localization using $^{57}$Co transmission source.

histologic measurements of tumor thickness in a total of 869 patients and showed a correlation coefficient of greater than 0.9 between the 2 methods and that adequate surgical margins were obtained based on US measurements in 72% of lesions. Less reliable results were obtained in thin tumors measuring less than 0.4 mm in thickness and in very thick tumors greater than 7.6 mm. US used in combination with fine-needle aspiration biopsy has also been used in detection of lymph node involvement in patients with melanoma, although its use has not yet been well established based on varying results. Bossi and colleagues[77] demonstrated in their study a sensitivity and specificity of 89.4% and 90.3%, respectively, using this method of lymphatic assessment, whereas Kahle and colleagues[78] were able to show that it was possible to demonstrate the localization of SNs successfully in 85% of patients. However, in a later study by Sanki and colleagues,[79] they were only able to demonstrate a 24.3% sensitivity in detection of SNs, with a resulting very high rate of false negatives.

The sensitivity of US in this setting has been shown to increase in high-risk patients, with higher Breslow thickness (>4 mm) and increased tumor volume (>1.00 mm$^3$), increasing the sensitivity in some studies to 76%.[80]

## LABORATORY TESTING

Evaluation of a patient's serum for prognostic biomarkers represents an easy, noninvasive, rapid, and potentially valuable method in the detection of disease burden, particularly in the early stages. Because of tumor biology and clinical heterogeneity of melanoma, tumor behavior, and thus prognosis, can vary significantly within the same stage of disease.[81] Thus, the investigation of biochemical serum markers is particularly important to determine the specific tumor profile in order to identify the behavior pattern of a particular patient's disease process to more accurately determine their level of disease burden, and overall treatment options and prognosis.

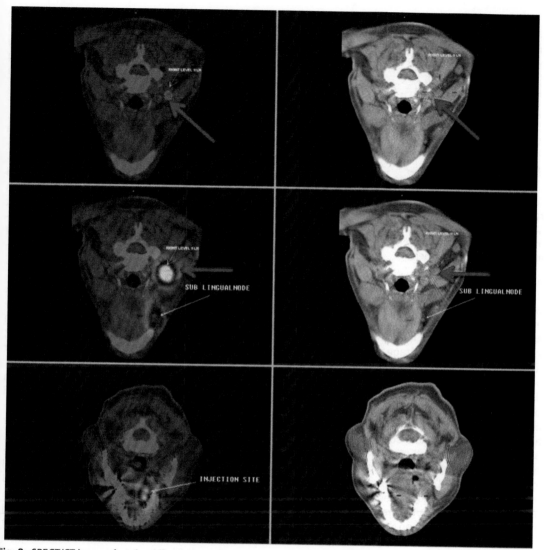

**Fig. 8.** SPECT/CT image showing injection site and lymph nodes in CT and fusion images. Red arrow demonstrates right level II cervical lymph node. Right sublingual lymph node and injection site are also represented in the picture.

An example of a serum biomarker for melanoma is lactate dehydrogenase (LDH), which, given the hypoxic environment of melanoma cells, catalyzes the conversion of pyruvate to lactate when oxygen levels are low. LDH does not represent a secreted enzyme, so an elevated serum level is thought to be secondary to spillage of the enzyme when melanoma cells outgrow their blood supply.[2] Despite the fact that it is not a specific marker for melanoma, the presence of elevated serum levels of this enzyme can be an indicator of distant metastasis in these patients. In a study of 121 melanoma patients by Finck and colleagues,[82] it was found that as an indicator of liver metastasis, the sensitivity and specificity of this biomarker in stage II patients were 95.1% and 82.8%, respectively, and 86.5% and 57.1% in stage III patients, respectively. Currently, LDH is the only serologic biomarker included in the American Joint Committee on Cancer staging system and is used to subclassify stage IV melanoma patients into an M1c category, which decreases the 1- and 2-year overall survival by about 50%.[83]

Another biomarker to receive some more recent attention is S100B, a small, acidic molecule involved in a variety of cellular functions, including tumor promotion, as it suppresses p53 function, and is part of the S100 molecule group, which is already recognized as a marker for melanoma tumors. Several studies have found that abnormally

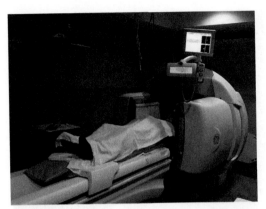

**Fig. 9.** SPECT-CT scanner with patient in position. Imaging duration can vary based on tracer drainage into the SN. Drainage pattern is visualized on the monitor above the scanner.

high levels of S100B in the serum of patients with melanoma are seen in disseminated disease, with Guo and colleagues[84] demonstrating its elevation in 73.9% of stage IV disease. In this same study, S100B was found to only be elevated in 1.3% and 8.7% of stage I and II patients, respectively, and thus does not represent a useful screening tool nor is it very useful in early detection. Increased levels of serum S100B have also been correlated to more aggressive disease profiles and resultant reduced survival.[85] In a meta-analysis by Mocellin and colleagues[86] including 3393 patients across all stages, they found that elevated S100B correlated with statistically significant poorer survival statistics and was found to be an independent prognostic factor at multivariate analysis. Moreover, another report demonstrated a direct correlation between S100B levels and Breslow tumor thickness, showing that a combined level of greater than 0.22 μg/L and Breslow thickness greater than 4 mm together had a sensitivity and specificity of 91% and 95%, respectively, for the presence of distant metastasis.[87] In a direct comparison of LDH and S100B by Wevers and colleagues,[88] they were able to show a correlation between disease-free survival and elevated S100B levels in patients with stage III melanoma, thus potentially representing a similar relationship as with LDH in stage IV patients, although S100B also has shown a relationship with elevated tumor burden in stage IV cases.[89] Unfortunately, given their poor sensitivity and specificity in stage I and II disease, they have limited use and value in early disease.

Cytokine profiles, both proinflammatory and anti-inflammatory, represent a valuable set of biomarkers that are easily accessed and measured and can aid in profiling tumors and their biologic behavior patterns. In a study examining 348 melanoma patients, Ortega-Martinez and colleagues[90] showed that serum levels of dermcidin (DCD) had prognostic value in patients with stage I and II melanoma, interestingly demonstrating that although DCD levels are elevated in patients with melanoma relative to healthy control subjects, patients with early disease who developed metastasis had a sharp decrease in levels of DCD, showing that patients with levels less than 2.98 μg/mL were more likely to develop metastasis. In the same study, they also examined vitronectin (VN) and found that patients with stage I and II disease with elevated levels of VN were 2.8 times more likely to develop metastasis, indicating that destruction of the basement membrane and extracellular matrix by tumor propagates the release of VN among other components into the serum, indicating potential metastatic activity.

Additional serum markers, such as IL-2 receptor, sICAM-1, IL-10, MIA, tyrosinase, VEGF, IL-6, and IL-8, to name a few, are currently being studied and have shown some relationship with advanced stage of disease and poor prognosis; however, they have yet to be further investigated.[91,92]

The liver represents one of the most common sites of metastasis of malignant melanoma and thus confers a poor prognosis and decreased survival. Assessment of liver enzyme levels and liver function tests, such as alkaline phosphatase, aspartate aminotransferase, alanine aminotransferase, gamma-glutamyl transpeptidase, and total bilirubin, can also be used in screening for and assessment of metastatic disease for the liver. This is well established in the monitoring of uveal melanoma, which shows levels rising at least 6 months before clinical detection of metastasis has occurred.[93] Despite this, measurement of serum liver enzymes and functional evaluation is not a part of the routine workup of metastatic melanoma.

## SUMMARY

Melanoma represents a devastating disease process with a relatively high mortality, and in which early detection and accurate staging are crucial in terms of prognosis. Unfortunately, diagnostic testing, such as advanced imaging and serum biomarkers, is currently inadequate for reliable identification of regional and distant metastasis, especially in early stages of the disease process and in routine surveillance. Fusion of some of the available imaging modalities and the combination of laboratory testing with certain tumor characteristics have resulted in improved detection rates; however, further research is needed to yield more reliable results, particularly in early-stage disease.

## CLINICS CARE POINTS

- When performing a diagnostic workup of a patient with melanoma, ensure the correct staging of the disease process, as this has a very significant impact on treatment and prognosis.
- Keep in mind that different imaging modalities are indicated based on site-specific evaluation in melanoma, and that use of more than one imaging technique may be indicated.
- Perform sentinel lymph node biopsy in conjunction with lymphoscintigraphy whenever possible, as this represents an excellent and well-proven modality in the assessment of regional lymph nodes.

## REFERENCES

1. Leiter U, Garbe C. Epidemiology of melanoma and nonmelanoma skin cancer—the role of sunlight. In: Reichrath J, editor. Sunlight, vitamin D and skin cancer. Advances in experimental medicine and biology. Basingstoke, UK: Springer Nature; 2008. p. 624.
2. Balch CM, Buzaid AC, Soong S, et al. Final version of the American Joint Committee on Cancer staging system for cutaneous melanoma. J Clin Oncol 2001; 19:3635–48.
3. Leiter U, Meier F, Schittek B. The natural course of cutaneous melanoma. J Surg Oncol 2004;86(4): 172–8.
4. Amer MH, Al-Sarraf M. Clinical presentation, natural history and prognostic factors in advanced malignant melanoma. Surg Gynecol Obstet 1979;149: 687–92.
5. Gromet MA, Ominsky SH, Epstein WL, et al. The thorax as the initial side for systemic relapse in malignant melanoma: a prospective survey of 324 patients. Cancer 1979;44:776–84.
6. Terhune MH, Swanson N, Johnson TM. Use of chest radiography in the initial evaluation of patients with localized melanoma. Arch Dermatol 1998;134: 569–72.
7. Huang CL, Provost N, Marghoob AA, et al. Laboratory tests and imaging studies in patients with cutaneous malignant melanoma. J Am Acad Dermatol 1998;39:451–63.
8. Webb WR, Gamsu G. Thoracic metastasis in malignant melanoma: a radiographic survey of 65 patients. Chest 1977;71:176–81.
9. Chen JTT Dahmash NS, Ravin CE. Metastatic melanoma to the thorax. AJR Am J Roentgenol 1981;137:293–8.
10. Libshitz HI, North LB. Pulmonary metastasis. Radiol Clin North Am 1982;20:437–51.
11. Heaston DK, Putman CE, Rodan BA, et al. Solitary pulmonary metastases in high-risk melanoma patients: a prospective comparison of conventional and computed tomography. AJR Am J Roentgenol 1983;141(1):169–74.
12. Silverman PM, Heaston DK, Korobkin M, et al. Computed tomography in the detection of abdominal metastasis from malignant melanoma. Invest Radiol 1984;19:309–12.
13. Zartman GM, Thomas MR, Robinson WA. Metastatic disease in patients with newly diagnosed malignant melanoma. J Surg Oncol 1987;35(3):163–4.
14. Buzaid AC, Tinoco L, Ross MI, et al. Role of computed tomography in the staging of patients with local-regional metastasis of melanoma. J Clin Oncol 1995;13:2104–8.
15. Paulsen SR, Huprich JE, Fletcher JG, et al. CT enterography as a diagnostic tool in evaluating small bowel disorders: review of clinical experience with over 700 cases. Radiographics 2006;26(3):641.
16. Blake SP, Weisinger K, Atkins MB, et al. Liver metastases from melanoma: detection with multiphasic contrast-enhanced CT. Radiology 1999;213(1):92.
17. Buzaid AC, Sandler AB, Mani S, et al. Role of computed tomography in the staging of primary melanoma. J Clin Oncol 1993;11(4):638–43.
18. Vilanova JC, Barcelo J. Diffusion-weighted whole-body MR screening. Eur J Radiol 2008;67:440–7.
19. Kwee TC, Takahara T, Ochiai R, et al. Diffusion-weighted whole-body imaging with background body signal suppression (DWIBS): features and potential application in oncology. Eur Radiol 2008;18:1937–52.
20. Gaviani ME, Mullins TA, Braga ET, et al. Improved detection of metastatic melanoma by T2-weighted imaging. AJNR Am J Neuroradiol 2006;27:605–8.
21. Mosav F, Gustav U, Hakan A. Whole-body MRI including diffusion-weighted imaging compared to CT for staging of malignant melanoma. Upsala J Med Sci 2013;118:91–7.
22. Davies MA, Liu P, McIntyre S. Prognostic factors for survival in melanoma patients with brain metastases. Cancer 2011;117(8):1687–96.
23. Kalkman E, Baxter G. Melanoma. Clin Radiol 2004; 59:313–26.
24. Coit DG, Thompson JA, Albertini MR. NCCN guidelines insights: melanoma - version 2.2018.
25. Tyler A, Janza B, Neskeya DM, et al. Is imaging of the brain necessary at diagnosis for cutaneous head and neck melanomas? Am J Otolaryngol 2018;39:631–5.

26. Ettl T, Irga S, Muller S. Value of anatomic site, histology and clinicopathological parameters for prediction of lymph node metastasis and overall survival in head and neck melanomas. J Craniomaxillofac Surg 2014;42(5):252–8.

27. Inamdar GS, Madhunapantula SV, Robertson GP. Targeting the MAPK pathway in melanoma: why some approaches succeed and other fail. Biochem Pharmacol 2010;80(5):624–37.

28. Hodis E, Watson IR, Kryukov GV. A landscape of driver mutations in melanoma. Cell 2012;150(2): 251–63.

29. Krauthammer M, Kong Y, Ha BH. Exome sequencing identifies recurrent somatic RAC1 mutations in melanoma. Nat Genet 2012;44(9):1006–14.

30. Son SH, Kang SM, Jeong SY. Prognostic value of volumetric parameters measured by pretreatment 18F FDG PET/CT in patients with cutaneous malignant melanoma. Clin Nucl Med 2016;41(6): e266–73.

31. Gulec SA, Faries MB, Lee CC, et al. The role of fluorine-18 deoxyglucose positron emission tomography in the management of patients with metastatic melanoma: impact on surgical decision making. Clin Nucl Med 2003;28(12):961–5.

32. Hindie E, Sarandi F, Banayan S. Nuclear medicine in early-stage melanoma: sentinel node biopsy-FDG-PET/CT. Pet Clin 2011;6:9–25.

33. Wagner JD, Schauwecker D, Davidson D. Prospective study of fluorodeoxyglucose-positron emission tomography imaging of lymph node basins in melanoma patients undergoing sentinel node biopsy. J Clin Oncol 1999;17:1508–15.

34. Schafer A, Herbst RA, Beiteke U. Sentinel lymph node excision (SLNE) and positron emission tomography in the staging of stage I-II melanoma patients. Hautarzt 2003;54:440–7.

35. Mijnhout GS, Hoekstra OS, van Lingen A. How morphometric analysis of metastatic load predicts the (un)usefulness of PET scanning: the case of lymph node staging in melanoma. J Clin Pathol 2003;56:283–6.

36. Longo MI, Lazaro P, Bueno C. Fluorodeoxyglucose-positron emission tomography imaging versus sentinel node biopsy in the primary staging of melanoma patients. Dermatol Surg 2003;29:245–8.

37. Hafner J, Schmid MH, Kempf W. Baseline staging in cutaneous malignant melanoma. Br J Dermatol 2004;150:677–86.

38. Havenga K, Cobben DC, Oyen WJ. Fluorodeoxyglucose-positron emission tomography and sentinel lymph node biopsy in staging primary cutaneous melanoma. Eur J Surg Oncol 2003;29:662–4.

39. Veit-Haibach P, Vogt FM, Jablonka R. Diagnostic accuracy of contrast-enhanced FDG-PET/CT in primary staging of cutaneous malignant melanoma. Eur J Nucl Med Mol Imaging 2009;36:910–8.

40. Wagner JD, Schauwecker DS, Davidson D, et al. FDG-PET sensitivity for melanoma lymph node metastases is dependent on tumor volume. J Surg Oncol 2001;77:237–42.

41. McIvor J, Siew T, Campbell A, et al. FDG PET in early stage cutaneous malignant melanoma. J Med Imag Rad Oncol 2014;58:149–54.

42. Reinhardt MJ, Joe AY, Jaeger U. Diagnostic performance of whole body dual modality 18F-FDG PET/CT imaging for N- and M-staging of malignant melanoma: experience with 250 consecutive patients. J Clin Oncol 2006;24:1178–87.

43. Krug B, Crott R, Lonneux M, et al. Role of PET in initial staging of cutaneous malignant melanoma: systematic review. Radiology 2008;249:836–44.

44. Pfannenberg C, Aschoff P, Schanza S, et al. Prospective comparison of 18F-fluorodeoxyglucose positron emission tomography/computed tomography and whole-body magnetic resonance imaging in staging of advanced malignant melanoma. Eur J Cancer 2007;43:557–64.

45. Schroer-Gunther MA, Wolff RF, Westwood ME. F-18-fluoro-2-deoxyglucose positron emission tomography (PET) and PET/computed tomography imaging in primary staging of patients with malignant melanoma: a systematic review. Syst Rev 2012;1:62.

46. Yancovitz M, Finelt N, Warycha MA. Role of radiologic imaging at the time of initial diagnosis of stage T1b-T3b melanoma. Cancer 2007;110:1107–14.

47. Constantinidou A, Hofman M, O'Doherty M, et al. Routine positron emission tomography and positron emission tomography/computed tomography in melanoma staging with positive sentinel node biopsy is of limited benefit. Melanoma Res 2008;18:56–60.

48. Strobel K, Dummer R, Husarik DB, et al. High-risk melanoma: accuracy of FDG PET/CT with added CT morphologic information for detection of metastases. Radiology 2007;244:566–74.

49. Strobel K, Skalsky J, Kalff V. Tumour assessment in advanced melanoma: value of FDG-PET/CT in patients with elevated serum S-100B. Eur J Nucl Med Mol Imaging 2007;34:1366–75.

50. Berzaczy D, Fueger B, Hoeller C, et al. Whole-body 18F-FDG-PET. MRI vs 18F-FDG-PET/CT in malignant melanoma. Mol Imaging Biol 2020;22:739–44.

51. Jouvet JC, Thomas L, Thomson V, et al. Whole-body MRI with diffusion-weighted sequences compared with 18 FDG PET-CT, CT and superficial lymph node ultrasonography in the staging of advanced cutaneous melanoma: a prospective study. J Eur Acad Dermatol Venereol 2014;28(2):176.

52. Schaarschmidt BM, Grueneisen J, Stebner V. Can integrated 18F-FDG PET/MR replace sentinel lymph node resection in malignant melanoma? Eur J Nucl Med Mol Imaging 2018;45(12):2093–102.

53. Testori A, De Salvo GL, Montesco MC. Clinical considerations on sentinel node biopsy in melanoma

from an Italian multicentric study on 1,313 patients (SOLISM-IMI). Ann Surg Oncol 2009;16(7):2018–27.

54. Marsden JR, Newton-Bishop JA, Burrows L. Revised UK guidelines for the management of cutaneous melanoma 2010. J Plast Reconstr Aesthet Surg 2010;63:1401–19.

55. Garbe C, Peris K, Hauschild A. Diagnosis and treatment of melanoma: European consensus-based interdisciplinary guideline. Eur J Cancer 2010;46: 270–83.

56. Morton DL, Thompson JF, Cochran AJ, et al, MSLT Group. Final trial report of sentinel-node biopsy versus nodal observation in melanoma. N Engl J Med 2014;370:599–609.

57. Yudd AP, Kepmf JS, Goydos JS, et al. Use of sentinel node lymphoscintigraphy in malignant melanoma. Radiographics 1999;19:343–53.

58. Uren RF, Howman-Giles RB, Thompson JF. Lymphatic drainage to triangular intermuscular space lymph nodes in melanoma on the back. J Nucl Med 1996;37:964–6.

59. Nieweg OE. False-negative sentinel node biopsy. Ann Surg Oncol 2009;16(8):2089–91.

60. Kaveh AH, Seminara NM, Barnes MA. Aberrant lymphatic drainage and risk for melanoma recurrence after negative sentinel node biopsy in middle-aged and older men. Head Neck 2016;38:754–60.

61. McMasters KM, Noyes RD, Reintgen DS. Lessons learned from the Sunbelt Melanoma Trial. J Surg Oncol 2004;86(4):212–23.

62. Miller MW, Vetto JT, Monroe MM, et al. False-negative sentinel lymph node biopsy in head and neck melanoma. Otolaryngol Head Neck Surg 2011; 145(4):606–11.

63. Chapman BC, Gleisner A, Kwak JJ. SPECT/CT improves detection of metastatic sentinel lymph nodes in patients with head and neck melanoma. Ann Surg Oncol 2016;23(8):2652–7.

64. Kwak JJ, Kesner AL, Gleisner A, et al. Utility of quantitative SPECT/CT lymphoscintigraphy in guiding sentinel lymph node biopsy in head and neck melanoma. Ann Surg Oncol 2020;27:1432–8.

65. Jimenez-Heffernan A, Ellmann A, Sado H. Results of a prospective multicenter International Atomic Energy Agency sentinel node trial on the value of SPECT/CT over planar imaging in various malignancies. J Nucl Med 2015;56(9):1338–44.

66. Quartuccio N, Garau LM, Arnone A, et al. Comparison of 99mTc-labeled colloid SPECT/CT and planar lymphoscintigraphy in sentinel lymph node detection in patients with melanoma: a meta-analysis. J Clin Med 2020;9:1680.

67. Thomsen JB, Sørensen JA, Grupe P, et al. Sentinel lymph node biopsy in oral cancer: validation of technique and clinical implications of added oblique planar lymphoscintigraphy and/or tomography. Eur J Nucl Med Mol Imaging 2009;36:1915–36.

68. Burton DA, Cashman JN. Allergic reaction to nano-colloid during lymphoscintigraphy for sentinel node biopsy. Br J Anaesth 2002;89:105.

69. Chicken DW, Mansouri R, Ell PJ, et al. Allergy to technetium-labeled nano colloidal albumin for sentinel node identification. Ann R Coll Surg Engl 2007;89:W12–3.

70. European Directorate for the Quality of Medicines. Technetium (99mTc) colloidal sulphur injection, European Pharmacopoeia. 5th ed. Strasbourg: EDQM, Council of Europe; 2005. p. 852.

71. United States Pharmacopeial Convention. Technetium (Tc-99m) sulfur colloid injection, United States Pharmacopeia 30. Rockville, MD: USP Convention; 2006. p. 3288.

72. Technetium-99m radiopharmaceuticals: manufacture of kits. Vienna: International Atomic Energy Agency; 2008.

73. Buscombe J, Paganelli G, Burak ZE, et al. Sentinel node in breast cancer procedural guidelines. Eur J Nucl Med Mol Imaging 2007;12:2154–9.

74. Waddington WA, Keshtgar MRS, Taylor I, et al. Radiation safety of the sentinel node technique in breast cancer. Eur J Nucl Med 2000;27:377–91.

75. Pandit-Tskar NN, Dauer LT, Montgomery L, et al. Organ and fetal absorbed dose estimates from Tc-99m-sulfur colloid lymphoscintigraphy and sentinel node localization in breast cancer patients. J Nucl Med 2006;47:1202–8.

76. Machet L, Belot V, Naori M, et al. Preoperative measurement of thickness of cutaneous melanoma using high-resolution 20 MHz ultrasound imaging: a monocenter prospective study and systematic review of the literature. Ultrasound Med Biol 2009;35(9): 1411–20.

77. Bossi MC, Sanvito S, Lovati E, et al. Role of high resolution color-Doppler US of the sentinel node in patients with stage I melanoma. Radiol Med 2001;102:357–62.

78. Kahle B, Hoffend J, Wacker J, et al. Preoperative ultrasonographic identification of the sentinel lymph node in patients with malignant melanoma. Cancer 2003;97:1947–54.

79. Sanki A, Uren RF, Moncrieff M. Targeted high-resolution ultrasound is not an effective substitute for sentinel lymph node biopsy in patients with primary cutaneous melanoma. J Clin Oncol 2009;27: 5614–9.

80. Voit CA, Gooskens SL, Siegel P. Ultrasound-guided fine-needle aspiration cytology as an addendum to sentinel lymph node biopsy can perfect the staging strategy in melanoma patients. Eur J Cancer 2014; 50:2280–8.

81. Gershenwald JE, Scolyer RA, Hess KR, et al. Melanoma staging: evidence-based changes in the American Joint Committee on Cancer eighth edition cancer staging manual. CA Cancer J Clin 2017;67: 472–92.

82. Finck SJ, Guiliano AE, Morton DL. LDH and melanoma. Cancer 1983;51(5):840–3.

83. Balch CM, Gershenwald JE, Soong SJ. Final version
of 2009 AJCC melanoma staging and classification.
J Clin Oncol 2009;27:6199–206.

84. Guo HB, Stoffel-Wagner B, Bierwirth T, et al. Clinical
significance of serum S100 in metastatic malignant
melanoma. Eur J Cancer 1995;31:1898–902.

85. von Schoultz E, Hansson LO, Djureen E. Prognostic
value of serum analyses of S-100 beta protein in malignant melanoma. Melanoma Res 1996;6:133–7.

86. Mocellin S, Zavagno G, Nitti D. The prognostic value
of serum S100B in patients with cutaneous melanoma: a meta-analysis. Int J Cancer 2008;123:
2370–6.

87. Abraha HD, Fuller LC, Du Vivier AW, et al. Serum
S-100 protein: a potentially useful prognostic marker
in cutaneous melanoma. Br J Dermatol 1997;137:
381–5.

88. Wevers KP, Krujiff S, Speijers MJ. S-100B: a stronger
prognostic biomarker than LDH in stage IIIB–C melanoma. Ann Surg Oncol 2013;20:2772–9.

89. Deckers EA, Kruijff S, Brouwers AH. The association
between active tumor volume, total lesion glycolysis
and levels of S-100B and LDH in stage IV melanoma
patients. Eur J Surg Oncol 2020;46:2147–53.

90. Ortega-Martinez I, Gardeazabal J, Erramuzpe A. Vitronectin and dermcidin serum levels predict the
metastatic progression of AJCC I-II early-stage melanoma. Int J Cancer 2016;139:1598–607.

91. Boyano MD, Garcia-Vasquez MD, Gardeazabal J.
Serum-soluble IL-2 receptor and IL-6 levels in patients with melanoma. Oncology 1997;54:400–6.

92. Garcia-Vasquez MD, Boyano MD, Canavate ML.
Interleukin-2 enhances the growth of human melanoma cells derived from primary but not from metastatic tumours. Eur Cytokine Netw 2000;11:654–61.

93. Kaiserman I, Amer R. Liver function tests in metastatic
uveal melanoma. Am J Ophthalmol 2004;137:236–43.

# Principles of Surgery in Head and Neck Cutaneous Melanoma

Srinivasa Rama Chandra, MD, BDS, FDSRCS (Eng), FIBCSOMS (Onc-Recon)[a],*,
Sravani Singu, BS[b], Jason Foster, MD[c]

## KEYWORDS

- Melanoma • Head and neck • Sentinel node • Wide local excision • Completion neck dissection
- Wide excision margin • Melanoma in situ • Nevus

## KEY POINTS

- Surgical excision is the primary treatment of early stage head and neck cutaneous melanomas.
- Head and neck melanoma more than 2 mm in depth needs a wide local excision with a 2 cm margin.
- A margin of more than 2 cm does not offer better overall survival or disease-free survival.
- Sentinel node biopsy is a consideration for head and neck melanomas exceeding 0.8 mm thickness/depth.
- Additional imaging modalities such as ultrasound and nuclear medicine–aided localization for sentinel node should be considered.
- After sentinel lymph node (SLN) excision, metastases to the sentinel node should be read and reviewed by a multidisciplinary tumor board, with at least 50 cases annually.

## INTRODUCTION

Melanoma is a heterogenetic entity. Close to 30% of cutaneous melanomas occur in the head and neck region. Five to twelve percent are hereditary with various mutation profiles. Lentigo maligna subtype may have a higher frequency of incidence in the head and neck, and surgical margin is more critical in these lesions with surrounding facial actinic changes. Currently, surgery is recommended for early stage melanomas (stages I and II) with immunotherapy options for advanced disease.

Antitumor immunity and molecular biology advancements have increased our understanding of this unique disease entity. Medical and surgical therapy evolution has involved multiple "trial and error" therapeutic interventional perspectives. Especially with lack of large-scale outcome studies and reviews, surgical resections and management

has been experimental in the last 200 years since the first case described in English by Norris.[1,2] Recognition of host immunity and targeted therapy with mono/combination immunotherapies is the current recommendation for reducing cytotoxicity, morbidity, and disease burden management. Sentinel lymph node mapping, dissection, and completion neck dissection are surgical aspects reviewed for their merits and indications.

## HISTORICAL PERSPECTIVE

Lack of historical perspective would condemn us to fatal errors. It is very accurate in the historical advances and experimentations with melanoma as a disease entity (**Table 1**). Surgical therapy for early stage and advanced melanoma management has evolved in the last decade compared with the previous 50 years. John Hunter described

[a] Oral and Maxillofacial Surgery, Oregon Health & Sciences University, 3181 SW Sam Jackson Park, Portland, OR 97239, USA; [b] University of Nebaraska Medical Center, College of Medicine, Omaha, NE 68198, USA; [c] Division of Surgical Oncology, University of Nebraska Medical Center, 986345 Nebraska Medical Center, Omaha, NE 68198-6345, USA
* Corresponding author.
E-mail address: chandrsr@ohsu.edu

Oral Maxillofacial Surg Clin N Am 34 (2022) 251–262
https://doi.org/10.1016/j.coms.2021.11.006

melanoma more than 200 years ago in 1787. The recognition of melanoma as a disease entity is attributed to Renée Laennec in 1812.[1] In 1969, Wallace Clark was the first to acknowledge heterogeneity in melanoma pathologically and the correlation of prognosis with the levels of invasion. The genetic heterogeneity among melanomas was finally detailed by Bastian in 2005.[1]

Clark's levels divided the depth of melanoma invasion between the dermis and subcutaneous fat by histologic and anatomic levels. Breslow classification system is based on a measured depth of invasion by millimeters. Breslow's is different from the anatomic compartments (Clark's), varying at various head and neck anatomic sites. Breslow depth is an independent predictor of patient outcome. Melanocytic markers are used to identify melanotic cells, and proliferative markers are currently used to identify tumor proliferation and mitotic figures.[2]

Head and neck melanoma surgical management involves

a. Optimal biopsy technique
b. Wide radial excision of the primary lesion or scar (wide local excision [WLE])
c. Sentinel lymph node biopsy (SLNB)
d. Parotid bed review and surgery
e. Complete lymph node dissection (CLND) and therapeutic neck Dissection
f. Immediate and definitive reconstruction

Every suspicious lesion as in **Fig. 1**, before biopsy of lesion and postbiopsy workup for definitive wide local excision, should be well illustrated and picture recorded in clinical notes. The radial excision margin is from the clinical edge or edge of biopsy scar of the lesion.

Surgery remains a therapy for curative intent in early stage and in situ disease.[3] Surgical excision of the localized lesion with clear margins has a 92% 5-year survival rate. Narrow excision is a 10 mm radial margin from the edge of the clinical lesion or residual scar. Less than 10 mm margin will achieve only 81% completion of resection. There is a definitive role for surgical management in advanced disease too. Complexity in head and neck lymphatic drainage and proximity to vital structures make WLE and SNLB difficult.[4] Previous excisions, scars, or altered lymphatics will change nodal drainage patterns.

The surgical guidelines and the surgeon's prerogative of the ideal margin, extent, and reconstructive timing and methods have been evolving with landmark publications and multicenter trials. Multicenter selective lymphadenectomy trials I and II (MSLT-I) and (MSLT-II), German Dermatologic Cooperative Oncology Group-selective lymphadenectomy trial (DeCOG-SLT), and few other randomized controlled trials exploring disease-free and overall survival outcomes are not head and neck–specific, but these have redirected disease management that has been extrapolated to head and neck melanoma surgical management too.[3–10]

## EARLY STAGE MELANOMA

Thin localized melanomas have the most significant surgical cure potential. The best independent predictor for cure istumor thickness and ulceration. The eighth edition of American Joint Committee on Cancer emphasizes these variables, including ulceration as a prognosticating factor.[5]

## SURGICAL BIOPSY TECHNIQUES AND MERITS

The diagnostic biopsy for a suspected head and neck melanoma should be able to accurately assess the thickness. The Breslow thickness is one of the most important prognostic factors for staging and surgical management. A palpable melanoma is perceived to be at least more than 1 mm thick.

The commonly encountered techniques of biopsy are shave biopsy, saucerization, and punch biopsies. There is no depth identification between a shave and saucerization (deeper) biopsy specimen.[8] A shave biopsy can be performed if the suspicion for invasive melanoma is low. This technique is a common dermatologic practice encountered. There is a risk of transection at anatomic junctional tissues such as the ear lobe with shave biopsies. Punch biopsies may be ideal and controlled for diameter and performed at the thickest portion of the primary lesion. Excisional biopsy without photographic or residual scar evidence of small lesions may be poor practice. Partial-thickness biopsy and transection may not be representative of thickness for diagnosis.

Excisional biopsy is appropriate with a 2 mm margin for definitive diagnosis. It is undertaken under local anesthesia in the outpatient setting.

### Surgical Excision and Staging

Definitive surgical excision is based on staging. Staging depends on a careful review of the pathology with the following complements.

1. Breslow thickness
2. argins of excision biomicroscopic examination
3. Mitotic rate per millimeters square (mitosis/$mm^2$)
4. Ulceration

**Table 1**
**Historical advances in melanoma: recognition and management**

| Pre-Columbian Mummy | Melanoma of Bone | ~ ~ ~2400 y Ago |
|---|---|---|
| Hippocrates of Cos | Black tumors | Fifth century |
| Drs Highmore and Bonet | Black tumors | 1651 |
| Henrici & Nothnagel | Fatal black tumors | 1757 |
| Hunter, John | Recognition of melanoma specimen of jaw (a fungus?) | 1787 |
| Laënnec, Renée | Description of melanoma as a disease entity | 1812 |
| Norris, William | Mole origin; hereditary nevi and melanoma correlation | 1820 |
| Cooper, Samuel | Description of surgical removal | 1840 |
| Snow, Herbert Lumley | Possible elective neck node excision | 1892 |
| Hadley, William Sampson | Wide local excision | 1907 |
| Krementz, Edward | Melphalan-isolated limb perfusion. First description | 1958 |
| Morton, Donald | Bacillus Calmette-Guerin (BCG) therapy for melanoma | 1968 |
| Gresser, Ion | Recognition of interferons for antitumor immunity | 1969 |
| **Clark, Wallace** | **Recognition of correlation of invasion to prognosis** | **1969** |
| **Breslow, Alexander** | **Relation between tumor thickness and prognosis** | **1970** |
| **Morton, Donald** | **First immunotherapy for metastatic cancer in humans; recognizes melanoma antigens; previously BCG vaccination** **Sentinel lymph node (SND) mapping technique** **Evidence of SND** | **1970 (immunotherapy)** **1974(Melanoma antigens)** **1992 (SND)** **2006** |
| AJCC | First staging for melanoma | 1988 |
| Davies, Helen | B-Raf mutation in melanoma | 2002 |
| Immunotherapy—advanced metastatic melanoma (FDA) | Pegylated interferons; ipilimumab; vemurafenib | 2011 |

*Abbreviation:* AJCC, The American Joint Committee on Cancer; FDA, Food and Drug Administration.

5. Vascular invasion, immunohistochemistry (IHC), in-transit metastasis, microsatellites, tumor-infiltrating lymphocytes, regression, desmoplasia, trophism, associated benign melanotic lesion, Soler Allis ptosis, predominant cell type, histologic growth pattern, growth phase and so forth

## PRIMARY MELANOMA EXCISION—WIDE LOCAL EXCISION

The principle of surgical excision is to eliminate by radial excision the "apparent" local primary lesion.

The excision margin is the "inapparent" adjacent area of tissue with the potential for residual or locoregional and distant spread. The lesion or scar edge as clinically evident with the margin for radial excision is undertaken to the depth of the deep fascia or anatomic transition. Excision deep to the subcutaneous fat or fascia is adequate.

There is a difference between trunk/extremity and head and neck lesion excision margins. In head and neck, for in situ lesions, the margin varies between 5 and 10 mm as circumferential margin of excision. But, clinical practice guidelines for the management of melanoma in Australia and New

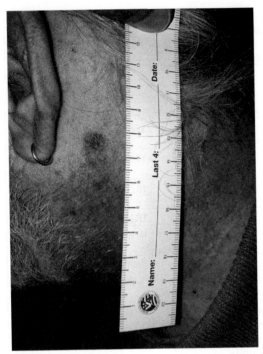

**Fig. 1.** Left postauricular suspicious lesion of head and neck region is documented before workup by biopsy and surgical planning.

Zealand have 5 mm as the margin for in situ lesions.[3–5,11]

Any excision should have consistent margins with vertical edges. Reexcision should be considered if the margin is less than appropriate for the defined thickness as soon as possible. Head and neck melanomas in the regions of significant actinic changes and presence of atypical melanocytes should be reviewed with additional immunohistochemical stains, multidisciplinary teams review with concordance.

The current recommendation for a thin lesion less than 2 mm thickness is an additional margin of 1 cm. More than 1 cm wide margin for the melanomas did not improve overall survival. For thick lesions of more than 2 mm thickness, a 1 cm margin is generally inadequate. There is ambiguity with very few studies for the ideal excision margins for lesions thicker than 4 mm. it is recognized as guidance of 2 cm margin for lesions more than 2 mm thick. Thicker melanomas and ulcerated lesions have a higher recurrence rate and poor survival.[12–15] Nodal deposit of tumor is higher with thicker melanomas (**Table 2**).

In randomized controlled trials of high-risk melanomas excision margin, Thomas and colleagues[13] retrospectively reviewed that 1 cm margin for melanomas at least (2 mm depth) is a greater risk of regional recurrence than 3 cm margin. But this 900 patient British study reported similar overall survival in both 1 cm and 3 cm excision margins in single melanomas of the trunk and extremities.[7–10,12,13,16–21] A Swedish study of 5 cm excision margins had a similar observation.[22]

## CRITICAL POINTS IN MARGIN EVALUATION

Inadequate margins potentiated locoregional recurrence and metastasis and increased mortality and morbidity. In transit, lesions increased recurrence too. Metastasis in melanoma is a continuum phenomenon with thicker or high-risk lesions. Frozen sections in thicker melanomas by hematoxylin and eosin staining are not sensitive or specific. IHC is standard of care since 1997, with HMB-45 and S100.

In-transit metastatic melanoma is any subcutaneous or skin tumor deposits that is more than 2 cm from the primary lesion. But the deposit should not be beyond the draining nodal basin regionally; this may be critical in head and neck lymphatic anatomic knowledge.

Anything that is within 2 cm from the primary tumor is termed "satellite metastasis." These are nonnodal locoregional metastases as a result of intralymphatic or probable angiotrophic spread of tumor cells. Microsatellites, in-transit and satellite, are part of "N" category in the eighth edition. As depicted in **Fig. 2**, the distances in head and neck of even the nodal basin are very close compared with the satellite lesion of extremities.

## SENTINEL LYMPH NODE BIOPSY

For head and neck melanoma lesions more than 0.8 mm in depth, the sentinel node should be identified, and a biopsy should be performed. SLNB is not recommended for melanoma in situ lesions. The rationale of SLNB is to identify the first dependent echelon drainage of the primary melanoma metastasis. If the drainage levels have no SLN positive disease, there is no metastatic disease. The sentinel node is not always the node closest or the "node of proximity" to the tumor. If the SLNB is positive, then further adjuvant therapy is rationalized, and the SLNB procedure provides locoregional control (reference). A positive SLNB also provides melanoma-specific survival (MSS) advantage as well as a clinical trial qualification. The status of the SLN is one of the critical factors in prognosis and in regard to recurrence (reference). Clinically palpable nodes can be subjected to fine-needle aspirate biopsy with or without ultrasound guidance with IHC review too. **Fig. 3** shows a computed tomography (CT) scan of the lesion

**Table 2**
**Surgical margins for cutaneous melanoma located on the head and neck**

| TNM Classification | Thickness | Total Margin |
|---|---|---|
| pTis | In situ | 5 mm–1 cm |
| pT1 | ≤1.0 mm | 1 cm |
| pT2 | 1.01–2.0 mm | 1–2 cm |
| pT3 | 2.01–4.0 mm | 2 cm |
| pT4 | ≥4.01 mm | 2 cm |

from the left mandibular border of the face with a radiolabeled dye injected.

The nuclear medicine imaging modality used to localize a sentinel node can cause a "shine through" with the radio labeled technetium-99 sulfur colloid dye injected intradermal in the vicinity to the tumor. So pre-WLE fine-cut CT scan and gamma probe post-WLE excision intraoperatively, as depicted in **Fig. 4**A, can be used to evaluate nodal basin after WLE.

Knowledge of head and neck angiolymphatic anatomy is essential for ideal identification and management of intraparotid and periparotid sentinel node. About 30% of SLN occurs in the parotid, where facial nerve injury is of significant concern. Large-volume referral centers are ideal than community-based dermatologic practices, as that is a learning curve regarding the identification and harvest of these sentinel nodes in the head and neck,[23] especially with a consistent, systematic pathologic handling of the SLN of smaller caliber. The SLNB guidelines are detailed in **Table 3**.

The node (N) criteria of melanoma staging include occult and clinically detected nodes. Clinically occult nodes were microscopic tumor deposit with or without radiographic evidence. The current practice is to apply investigative modalities such as ultrasound or other radiographic modalities for "clinical detection." **Figs. 3** and **4**, and **Figs. 5–7**, all illustrate detection of a potential nodal activity.

Based on the MSLT and the DeCOG multicenter trials[6–8] and guidelines, it is suggested that positive sentinel node metastasis can be followed with nodal observation with ultrasonography.[6–9] Based on these trials, a CLND did not offer superior survival rates compared with nodal observation with ultrasonography. There is a higher incidence of false-negative rate for nodal recurrence among head and neck melanomas. And there is an increased frequency of interval node and false-negative rate in head and neck melanomas as in comparison to the trunk and extremity.[23] But a positive head and neck sentinel node has a high predictive value for recurrence.[19] In both thin and thick melanomas, with a positive sentinel node, the prognosis is poor.[19,24,25] Multiple systematic reviews inclusive of 267 reviewed cases with 85% negative SLN harvest was independent of primary head and neck subsite and drainage.[19–21,23,24] A negative SLN biopsy did not portend poor survival when compared with a positive initial SLN.

Current guidelines for follow-up after sentinel node biopsy and excision is nodal observation with an ultrasound scan. CLND may not be considered due to the significant morbidity of lymphedema and associated morbidity of neck dissection with limited overall survival benefit.

## Parotid and Parotid Region Sentinel Lymph Node Biopsy

### Illustration of parotid dissection
About 30% of SLN occurs in the Parotid, where facial nerve injury is of significant concern.[26] So the authors' clinical practice is in the use of continuous facial nerve monitoring as shown with blue, red, and purple leads in the illustration of right cheek melanoma excision and SLNB (**Fig. 6**A and the parotid bed dissection in **6B**.).[26] There is a high incidence of nodal drainage to the parotid from head and neck melanomas. Parotid SLNs are broadly classified with a node superficial to parotid glandular structure (adherent or embedded) versus a deep intraglandular node, single or multiple.

The parotid nodes are small and in the range of 3 to 6 mm in size. They can be multiple, and

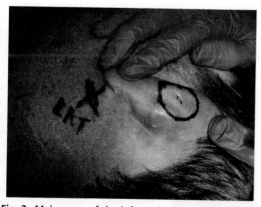

**Fig. 2.** Melanoma of the left ear helix with the biopsy scar identified and a wide local excision planned with the circular skin mark. The identified lateral sentinel lymph node of the ipsilateral neck is preoperatively identified and marked.

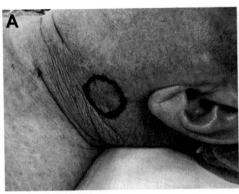
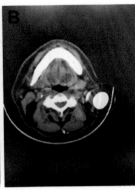

Fig. 3. A) Left mandibular biopsy scar of the biopsy-proven melanoma. (B) The nuclear medicine imaging modality used to localize a sentinel node can cause a "shine through" with the radiolabeled technetium-99 sulfur colloid dye injected intradermal in the vicinity to the tumor. So pre-WLE fine-cut CT scan and gamma probe post-WLE excision intraoperatively, as depicted in Fig. 4A, can be used to evaluate nodal basin after WLE.

lymphoscintigraphy and intraoperative gamma probe occasionally produce a "shine through effect," a stacked nodal effect with a mass shine on imaging. Resolution of single-photon emission CT may be limited if not well localized in delineating the parotid nodes. Morbidity of facial nerve traction or direct injury has been encountered in SLNB parotid dissection. Some centers advocate superficial parotidectomy with lower nerve morbidity as primary nerve identification and monitoring in the management of intraparotid SLNs. Preoperative imaging and review of all aspects of WLE, parotid excision, and SLNB with nerve anatomy are essential discussion highlights for consent with patients and neuromuscular relaxation with anesthesiologists.

### Neck Dissection—Complete Lymph Node Dissection and Therapeutic Node Dissection

#### Neck dissection illustration
Scalp and periauricular melanomas can drain to levels II to V, parotid, occipital, or periauricular bed of lymph nodes (see Fig. 7). Anterior scalp or vertex drainage can be discordant or concordant to the laterality. Most often, they drain to I to IV levels. SLNB is mapped, and then nodal excision is performed after the primary and margins are excised in the same operation. So, the parotid bed and overlapping intraoperative localization can be precise. Revisit resections and therapeutic NDs are selective and functional NDs, sparing all vital structures as illustrated in Fig. 7. Immunotherapy as an adjunct is always a consideration before aggressive CLND or salvage node dissection. So, morbidity of significant lymphedema, nerve injury, and so forth are mitigated. But in cases where there is extensive metastatic tumor deposit or patient's poor compliance for surveillance, node dissection may be undertaken. Lack of access to ultrasound is another potential consideration.[26,27]

**Surgical options in metastatic melanoma of head and neck primary lesions** In patients with advanced metastatic disease or in-transit lesions, resection of the additional metastatic lesion can be considered in addition to immunotherapy, only if negative margins can be surgically achieved.

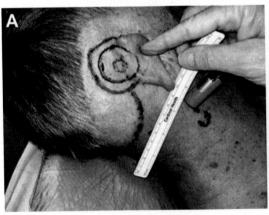
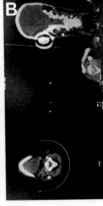

Fig. 4. A) The patient with a biopsy-proven postauricular melanoma with radial margins drawn and the gamma probe being used for detection intraoperatively of the node with the uptake of the radioactive dye. (B) The SPECT-CT scan in axial image on the left and the coronal section on the right with hot uptake of the radiolabeled injection. SPECT, single-photon emission computed tomography.

**Table 3**
Sentinel lymph node biopsy guidelines

| TNM Classification | Thickness | Sentinel Lymph Node Biopsy | Merits |
|---|---|---|---|
| pTis | *Melanoma in situ* | Not recommended<br>Advanced imaging may be considered | Review final pathology<br>Lentigo maligna |
| pT1 | ≤1.0 mm | Primary melanoma > 0.8 mm thick<br>SLNB may be considered<br>Clark level 4 or 5<br>Microstaging high mitotic rate (≥1 mitosis/mm²),<br>Uceration or microsatellites | MSS benefit;<br>adjuvant therapy &/or clinical trial |
| pT2 and pT3 | 1.01–2.0 mm<br>Thin<br><br>Thick<br>2.01–4.0 mm | SLNB strongly recommended<br>Same operation as WLE<br>Microstaging | Locoregional control<br>MSS benefit;<br>adjuvant therapy &/or clinical trial |
| pT4 | ≥4.01 mm | SLNB strongly recommended<br>Same operation as WLE<br>Advanced SLN mapping<br>metastatic workup | Locoregional control<br>MSS benefit;<br>adjuvant therapy &/or clinical trial |

Sentinel lymph node biopsy (SLNB) for cutaneous melanoma located on the head and neck.

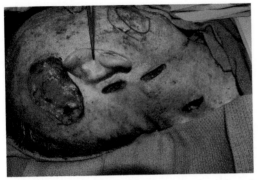

**Fig. 5.** An intraoperative WLE excision of a left scalp lesion with 3 right neck SNBs performed.

Completion resection in such cases may not be preferred other than for in-transit and confined satellite metastases. Palliative consideration for surgery may be done on a case-by-case basis with the review of systemic therapies involving BRAF, MEK, anti-CTLA4, and programmed cell death protein 1 inhibitors.[10,28] Adverse effects with endocrinopathies, wound healing, and so forth are to be reviewed with the patient, with multiple case reports published.[29]

### Oncological Surveillance for Head and Neck Melanoma

The nodal follow-up currently as recommended is highlighted in **Table 4**: clinical examination with an ultrasound scan, 4- to 6-month interval for the first 2 years, and 6-/2-/12-month interval for the third to fifth years.[10]

## CONTROVERSIES

Most of the current surgical guidelines are for those aged 18 years and older. There are sizable melanotic nevus and associated malignant lesions with no guidance on management. It is well known that lymphatic drainage is variable in head and neck regions. Any previous procedures or radiation make the nodal draining more exponentially unpredictable.[24,30]

### Reduced Excision Margins in Head and Neck Critical Areas

Excision margins and recommendations are currently based on a retrospective review of data from less than a dozen cohorts.

In head and neck anatomic subsites, wide excision margins for primary eradication of apparent and inapparent melanoma may not be possible. Occasionally, even if the subsite allows for such large excisions, the morbidity and reconstructive effort do not increase overall survival. A prospect cohort of 79 cases of head and neck melanomas in close proximity to eye, nose, ear, and the mouth were reviewed with the reduced excision margins versus guideline-based WLE. This reduced excision margins in the head and neck areas did not increase local recurrence rates.[21] Forty-two of the seventy-nine patient cohort had reduced margins of 0.5 cm for lesions less than 1 mm thick, 0.5 to 1.0 cm for lesions 1.01 to 2.0 mm thick, and 1.0 cm margin for greater than 2.0 cm thick melanomas. In a follow up of more than 5 years the recurrence free survival by margin reduction in critical area lesion excision of head and neck melanomas was 91.9%, compared with 90.4% of regular WLE guidelines based resection. The overall recurrence rate in this study was 8.9%.

In another study in an Australian patient group with thicker melanomas of more than 4 mm of head and neck including scalp, periauricular regions along with critical areas of the face by Ruskin and colleagues, identified wider margins did not significantly improve locoregional recurrence.[15,26,27,31,32]

Subclinical extensions in all lentigo maligna, melanoma in situ, and invasive melanoma in the head and neck are known beyond the 5 mm and further studies show in extension of greater than 10 mm. But clinical specialties and regional

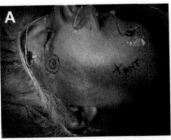
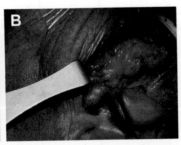
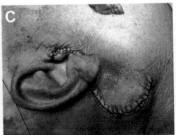

**Fig. 6.** (A) Continuous facial nerve monitor is used with implanted leads. (B) Traditional parotid approach and superficial gland resection with the identified multiple nodes is a low morbid procedure. (C) Postparotid dissection and closure.

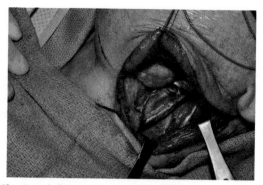

**Fig. 7.** A left selective neck dissection with posterior retraction of sternomastoid muscle exhibiting the spinal accessory nerve. The internal jugular and carotid vessels are noted in the well of the picture with digastric muscle and submandibular gland in the anterior-superior position.

confusion are present in classifying in situ and lentigo maligna by terminology and classification.[11,31–33]

Based on at least 6 randomized controlled trials, the American Academy of Dermatology, and National Comprehensive Cancer Network Practice Guidelines (NCCN) guidelines[11,14,15,26,27,31,32] recommending 10 mm margin for invasive melanoma, only 16 had head and neck patient cohorts out of 4231 invasive melanomas.[6] The reported eradicated rate with 10 mm margin in head and neck melanomas was between 52% and 91%.[15,26]

### Elective Neck Dissection

McDonald and colleagues[25] noted in a negative SLN biopsy did not portend poor survival compared with positive initial SLN.

## SURGICAL GUIDELINES FOR HEAD AND NECK MELANOMA MANAGEMENT
### Regional and Medical-Surgical Specialty Variations in the Surgical Management

There is a lack of level I evidence and literature regarding head and neck melanoma management in screening, margin resection in critical areas, completion of neck dissection, systemic immunotherapies, and follow-up protocol.

Australian cancer network (Australia and New Zealand), Cancer care Ontario and Canadian Medical Association (Canada), European Society for Medical Oncology (Europe), NCCN (United States),and directory of cancer guidelines are the 5 acclaimed recommendation groups for updated guidance. There are variations and differences in recommendations for surgical margins between the Australian and the other 3 groups.[11,22,34–37]

**Table 4**
**Current list of guidelines for Sentinel Lymph Node Biopsy (SLNB)**

| Guidelines | Year |
|---|---|
| National Comprehensive Cancer Network Practice Guidelines (NCCN) | 2017 |
| "In general, SLNB is not recommended for primary melanoma <0.75 mm thick. For melanomas, 0.76–1.00 mm, SLNB may be considered in the appropriate clinical context" | — |
| National Institute of Clinical Excellence (NICE) | 2015 |
| Morton D, Cochran A, Thompson J, Elashoff R, Essner R, Glass E, et al. Multicenter Selective Lymphadenectomy Trial Group: Sentinel node biopsy for early-stage melanoma: Accuracy and morbidity in MSLT-I, an international multicenter trial. Ann Surg. 2005;242(3):302–11 | — |
| "Do not offer imaging or sentinel lymph node biopsy to people who have stage IA melanoma or those who have stage IB melanoma with a Breslow thickness of 1 mm or less." | — |
| American Society of Clinical Oncology and Society of Surgical Oncology Joint Clinical Practice Guideline (ASCO/SSO) | 2012 |
| Rousseau DL, Ross MI, Johnson MM, Prieto VG, Lee JE, Mansfield PF, et al. Revised American Joint Committee on Cancer staging criteria accurately predict sentinel lymph node positivity in clinically node-negative melanoma patients. Ann Surg Oncol. 2003;10(5):569–74. | — |
| "Available evidence does not support routine SLN biopsy for patients with melanomas that are T1 or | — |

(continued on next page)

| Table 4 (continued) | |
|---|---|
| **Guidelines** | **Year** |
| <1 mm Breslow thickness although it may be considered in selected high-risk cases." | |
| Such high-risk factors may include Breslow thickness >0.75 mm, ulceration, or mitoses $\geq 1/$ mm$^2$ | — |
| European Society for Medical Oncology (ESMO) | 2012 |
| Valsecchi ME, Silbermins D, de Rosa N, Wong SL, Lyman GH. Lymphatic mapping and sentinel lymph node biopsy in patients with melanoma: A meta-analysis. J Clin Oncol. 2011;29(11):1479–87. | — |
| "SLN biopsy should be performed for tumor thickness of >1 mm and/or ulceration" | — |

*Adapted from* Joyce KM. Surgical Management of Melanoma. In: Ward WH, Farma JM, editors. Cutaneous Melanoma: Etiology and Therapy [Internet]. Brisbane (AU): Codon Publications; 2017 Dec 21. Chapter 7. Available from: https://www.ncbi.nlm.nih.gov/books/NBK481850/. *Reprinted* with permission of Dr. Kenneth M. Joyce.

## *Mohs Versus Conventional Margin Clearance*

It is unsettled with regard to whether Mohs or conventional margin clearance has better disease-free survival, overall survival, and MSS, especially with melanomas in critical areas of the face around the periocular, periauricular, and perioral adnexal regions.[30] Parotid and parotid lymph nodes are fairly small and occasionally in close proximity to facial nerve. Interval lymph nodes in this region are a challenge to harvest and an occasional diagnostic injection can display nodes as overlap with shine-through effect and pose challenge in excison and diagnosis. A single operative appointment in the primary lesion excision, as well as the sentinel lymph node dissection has shown to be more accurate.[30]

## MUCOSAL MELANOMA OF THE HEAD AND NECK

Malignant mucosal melanoma of the head and neck is an extensive topic by itself. This mucosal variant of the head and neck version is prone to significant distant metastasis and death even with adequate margin clearance. The head and neck subsites of sinonasal compared with oral have no demonstrated statistically significant difference in overall outcomes. All the subsites are amenable to surgery, followed by consideration for systemic immunotherapies. Nodal staging and management are part of surgical therapy. There are very few large cohort trials for guidance in treatment.

## SUMMARY

The critical long-term survival variables in head and neck melanomas are age, the thickness of invasion, ulceration, sentinel lymph node positivity, and history.

## CLINICS CARE POINTS

- When a patient has a new diagnosis of melanoma, assess tumor thickness and ulceration, as they are the best independent predictors for cure.
- When the diagnosis is early stage melanoma (stage I or II), surgery with immunotherapy is recommended.
- If suspicion for invasive melanoma is low, then a shave biopsy can be done.
- When doing an excisional biopsy, a 2 mm margin is necessary for definitive diagnosis.
- When doing WLE for in situ melanoma, margins should be 5 to 10 mm circumferentially.
- When doing WLE for lesions less than or equal to 1 mm in thickness, margins should be 1 cm circumferentially.
- When doing WLE for lesions greater than 1.01 mm and less than 2 mm in thickness, margins should be 1 to 2 cm circumferentially.
- When doing WLE for lesions greater than 2.01 mm and less than 4 mm in thickness, margins should be 2 cm circumferentially.
- When doing WLE for lesions greater than 4.01 mm in thickness, margins should be 2 cm circumferentially.
- If a head and neck melanoma is more than 0.8 mm in depth, consider doing an SLNB.
- If sentinel node metastasis is positive, then consider nodal observation with ultrasonography, as positivity indicates high predictive value for recurrence.

- If lack of ultrasonography in cases where sentinel node is positive, consider therapeutic node dissection.
- For management of intraparotid SLNs, some institutions advocate superficial parotidectomy with lower nerve morbidity.
- If margins of head and neck melanomas are imperceptible and melanoma is not thick nor invasive, then consider Mohs surgery; this excludes parotid and anatomically critical areas of the eye.

## REFERENCES

1. Lee C, Collichio F, Ollila D, et al. Historical review of melanoma treatment and outcomes. Clin Dermatol 2013;31(2):141–7.
2. Davis LE, Shalin SC, Tackett AJ. Current state of melanoma diagnosis and treatment. Cancer Biol Ther 2019;20(11):1366–79.
3. Ward WH, Farma JM, editors. Cutaneous melanoma: etiology and therapy [internet]. Brisbane (AU): Codon Publications; 2017.
4. Gardner LJ, Strunck JL, Wu YP, et al. Current controversies in early-stage melanoma: questions on incidence, screening, and histologic regression. J Am Acad Dermatol 2019;80(1):1–12.
5. Gershenwald JE, Scolyer RA, Hess KR, et al, for members of the American Joint Committee on Cancer Melanoma Expert Panel and the International Melanoma Database and Discovery Platform. Melanoma staging: evidence-based changes in the American Joint Committee on Cancer eighth edition cancer staging manual. CA Cancer J Clin 2017; 67(6):472–92.
6. Bello DM, Faries MB. The landmark series: MSLT-1, MSLT-2 and DeCOG (management of lymph nodes). Ann Surg Oncol 2020;27(1):15–21.
7. Morton DL, Thompson JF, Essner R, et al. Validation of the accuracy of intraoperative lymphatic mapping and sentinel lymphadenectomy for early-stage melanoma: a multicenter trial. Multicenter Selective Lymphadenectomy Trial Group. Ann Surg 1999; 230(4):453–63. discussion 463–5.
8. Morton DL, Cochran AJ, Thompson JF, et al, Multicenter Selective Lymphadenectomy Trial Group. Sentinel node biopsy for early-stage melanoma: accuracy and morbidity in MSLT-I, an international multicenter trial. Ann Surg 2005;242(3):302–11. ; discussion 311–3.
9. Krown SE, Chapman PB. Defining adequate surgery for primary melanoma. N Engl J Med 2004;350(8): 823–5.
10. Wright FC, Souter LH, Kellett S, et al, Melanoma Disease Site Group. Primary excision margins, sentinel lymph node biopsy, and completion lymph node dissection in cutaneous melanoma: a clinical practice guideline. Curr Oncol 2019;26(4):e541–50.
11. Kunishige JH, Doan L, Brodland DG, et al. Comparison of surgical margins for lentigo maligna versus melanoma in situ. J Am Acad Dermatol 2019;81(1): 204–12.
12. Faries MB, Thompson JF, Cochran AJ, et al. Completion dissection or observation for sentinel-node metastasis in melanoma. N Engl J Med 2017; 376(23):2211–22.
13. Thomas JM, Newton-Bishop J, A'Hern R, et al, United Kingdom Melanoma Study Group; British Association of Plastic Surgeons; Scottish Cancer Therapy Network. Excision margins in high-risk malignant melanoma. N Engl J Med 2004;350(8): 757–66.
14. Fong ZV, Tanabe KK. Comparison of melanoma guidelines in the U.S.A., Canada, Europe, Australia and New Zealand: a critical appraisal and comprehensive review. Br J Dermatol 2014; 170(1):20–30.
15. Moyer JS, Rudy S, Boonstra PS, et al. Efficacy of staged excision with permanent section margin control for cutaneous head and neck melanoma. JAMA Dermatol 2017;153(3):282–8.
16. Morton DL, Thompson JF, Cochran AJ, et al, MSLT Group. Final trial report of sentinel-node biopsy versus nodal observation in melanoma. N Engl J Med 2014;370(7):599–609.
17. Leiter U, Stadler R, Mauch C, et al, German Dermatologic Cooperative Oncology Group. Final analysis of DeCOG-SLT trial: no survival benefit for complete lymph node dissection in patients with melanoma with positive sentinel node. J Clin Oncol 2019; 37(32):3000–8.
18. Fisher SR. Elective, therapeutic, and delayed lymph node dissection for malignant melanoma of the head and neck: analysis of 1444 patients from 1970 to 1998. Laryngoscope 2002;112(1):99–110.
19. de Rosa N, Lyman GH, Silbermins D, et al. Sentinel node biopsy for head and neck melanoma: a systematic review. Otolaryngol Head Neck Surg 2011; 145(3):375–82.
20. Teng J, Halbert T, McMurry TL, et al. Histopathologic margin distance in survival in resection of cutaneous melanoma of the head and neck. Laryngoscope 2015;125(8):1856–60.
21. Rawlani R, Rawlani V, Qureshi HA, et al. Reducing margins of wide local excision in head and neck melanoma for function and cosmesis: 5-year local recurrence-free survival. J Surg Oncol 2015;111(7): 795–9.
22. Cohn-Cedermark G, Rutqvist LE, Andersson R, et al. Long term results of a randomized study by the Swedish Melanoma Study Group on 2-cm versus 5-cm resection margins for patients with cutaneous

melanoma with a tumor thickness of 0.8-2.0 mm. Cancer 2000;89:1495–501.

23. Giudice G, Leuzzi S, Robusto F, et al. Sentinel lymph node biopsy in head and neck melanoma*. G Chir 2014;35(5–6):149–55.

24. Ruskin O, Sanelli A, Herschtal A, et al. Excision margins and sentinel lymph node status as prognostic factors in thick melanoma of the head and neck: a retrospective analysis. Head Neck 2016;38(9):1373–9.

25. McDonald K, Page AJ, Jordan SW, et al. Analysis of regional recurrence after negative sentinel lymph node biopsy for head and neck melanoma. Head Neck 2013;35(5):667–71.

26. O'Brien CJ, Coates AS, Petersen-Schaefer K, et al. Experience with 998 cutaneous melanomas of the head and neck over 30 years. Am J Surg 1991;162:310–4.

27. Balch CM, Soong SJ, Smith T, et al. Long-term results of a prospective surgical trial comparing 2 cm vs. 4 cm excision margins for 740 patients with 1-4 mm melanomas. Ann Surg Oncol 2001;8:101–8.

28. Lee JJ, Lian CG. Molecular testing for cutaneous melanoma: an update and review. Arch Pathol Lab Med 2019;143(7):811–20.

29. Wang DY, Salem JE, Cohen JV, et al. Fatal toxic effects associated with immune checkpoint inhibitors: a systematic review and meta-analysis. JAMA Oncol 2018;4(12):1721–8. Erratum in: JAMA Oncol. 2018 Dec 1;4(12):1792.

30. Gannon CJ, Rousseau DL Jr, Ross MI, et al. Accuracy of lymphatic mapping and sentinel lymph node biopsy after previous wide local excision in patients with primary melanoma. Cancer 2006;107(11):2647–52.

31. Wilson JB, Walling HW, Scupham RK, et al. Staged excision for lentigo maligna and lentigo maligna melanoma: analysis of surgical margins and long-term recurrence in 68 cases from a single practice. J Clin Aesthet Dermatol 2016;9:25–30.

32. Mangold AR, Skinner R, Dueck AC, et al. Risk factors predicting positive margins at primary wide local excision of cutaneous melanoma. Dermatol Surg 2016;42:646–52.

33. Valentin-Noguras SM, Brodland DG, Zitelli JA, et al. Mohs micrographic surgery using MART-1 immunostain in the treatment of invasive melanoma and melanoma in situ. Dermatol Surg 2016;42:733–44.

34. Veronesi U, Cascinelli N. Narrow excision (1-cm margin): a safe procedure for thin cutaneous melanoma. Arch Surg 1991;126:438–41.

35. Khayat D, Rixe O, Martin G, et al. Surgical margins in cutaneous melanoma (2 cm versus 5 cm for lesions measuring less than 2.1-mm thick): long-term results of a large European multicentric phase III study. Cancer 2003;97:1941–6.

36. Gillgren P, Drzewiecki KT, Niin M, et al. 2-cm versus 4-cm surgical excision margins for primary cutaneous melanoma thicker than 2 mm: a randomised, multicentre trial. Lancet 2011;378:1635–42.

37. Hayes AJ, Maynard L, Coombes G, et al. Wide versus narrow excision margins for high-risk, primary cutaneous melanomas: long-term follow-up of survival in a randomised trial. Lancet Oncol 2016;17:184–92.

# Mohs Micrographic Surgery for the Treatment of Cutaneous Melanomas of the Head and Neck

Emilie S. Jacobsen, MD[a,b], Teo Soleymani, MD, FAAD, FACMS[a,c],*

## KEYWORDS

- Melanoma • Mohs micrographic surgery • Wide local excision • Immunostain • MART-1
- Oncology • Surgery • Reconstruction

## KEY POINTS

- Historically, the standard of care for management of melanoma in any anatomic location has been conventional wide local excision (WLE) with predetermined clinical surgical margins.
- No randomized controlled trial has demonstrated a difference in local recurrence, nodal metastases, or disease-specific death favoring wide versus narrow surgical excision margins using traditional WLE, indicating that tumor thickness and width of clinical surgical margins are not directly correlative.
- Melanomas of the head and neck, particularly those arising in chronically sun-damaged skin, often demonstrate extensive and asymmetric subclinical extension, which increases the risk of upstaging, local recurrence, and need for complex reconstruction after conventional excision.
- Traditional WLE using standard vertical section "breadloaf" pathologic processing allows for limited histopathologic margin assessment; in many instances, less than 1% of the true surgical margin is evaluated, whereas Mohs micrographic surgery allows for complete circumferential peripheral and deep margin assessment yielding histopathologic evaluation of 100% of the true surgical margin.
- For melanomas of the head and neck, particularly those arising in chronically sun-damaged skin, tumor extirpation with Mohs micrographic surgery using intraoperative immunohistochemical staining offers superior, durable tumor control and improved overall survival.

## INTRODUCTION

Surgical excision has long been the mainstay of treatment of primary cutaneous melanoma. Historically, the standard of care for management of melanoma in any anatomic location has been conventional wide local excision (WLE) with prescribed clinically defined surgical excision margins based on the Breslow depth of the tumor. Importantly, traditional WLE allows for very limited histopathological evaluation of the true surgical margin; in fact, standard vertical section "breadloaf" pathology examines less than 1% of the true surgical margin. Logically, the risk of residually positive margins or local recurrence is high when using traditional WLE. As such, to account

[a] Division of Dermatologic Surgery, David Geffen School of Medicine at University of California Los Angeles, 10833 Le Conte Ave, Los Angeles, CA 90095, USA; [b] Division of Dermatology, David Geffen School of Medicine, University of California, Los Angeles, Los Angeles, CA 90095, USA; [c] Mohs Micrographic and Reconstructive Surgery, Dermatologic Oncology, Pigmented Lesion and Melanoma Clinic, David Geffen School of Medicine, University of California, Los Angeles, Los Angeles, CA 90095, USA
* Corresponding author. Mohs Micrographic and Reconstructive Surgery, Dermatologic Oncology, Pigmented Lesion and Melanoma Clinic, David Geffen School of Medicine, University of California, Los Angeles, Los Angeles, CA 90095.
E-mail address: tsoleymani@mednet.ucla.edu

Oral Maxillofacial Surg Clin N Am 34 (2022) 263–271
https://doi.org/10.1016/j.coms.2021.11.005
1042-3699/22/© 2021 Elsevier Inc. All rights reserved.

for this limitation in margin assessment, broad (and somewhat arbitrary) clinical margins have been studied and defined, based on a perpetuating dogma that "if you cast a wide enough [surgical] net," you may catch "local microsatellites" and thus somehow affect the metastatic process. However, to date, there has not been a single randomized controlled trial (RCT) demonstrating a difference in local recurrence, nodal metastases, or disease-specific death favoring those undergoing wide versus narrow surgical excision margins using traditional WLE, indicating that tumor thickness and width of clinical surgical margins are not directly correlative.

Importantly, cutaneous melanomas of the head and neck, particularly those that arise in chronically sun-damaged skin, often demonstrate extensive asymmetric subclinical extension.

Although Mohs micrographic surgery (MMS) has long been established as the gold standard for treatment of nonmelanoma skin cancers with markedly superior cure rates and lower rates of local recurrence, regional nodal metastases, and death, melanoma management has been slow to adapt and continues to use arbitrary clinical margins based on histopathologic tumor thickness, regardless of the understanding that standard vertical-section pathology examines less than 1% of the true margin.

With recent advances in MMS and the advent of precise, highly specialized intraoperative immunohistochemical stains resulting in superior tumor cure rates, paradigms in treatment philosophy and management are rightfully shifting. This article reviews the management of primary cutaneous melanomas of the head and neck with MMS and highlights the expanding body of evidence supporting its use.

### Historical Perspectives and Background

Surgical treatment of primary cutaneous melanoma historically has been based on the concept of WLE to capture spread of atypical melanocytes. This technique involves the excision of clinically visible tumor along with a clinical margin of normal-appearing skin. The initial defining creed set out in the early 1900s consisted of a standard radical 5-cm margin around the primary tumor, based on the experience of British surgeon William Sampson Handley, who stated in 1907: "The process of dissemination in malignant melanoma is primarily one of centrifugal lymphatic permeation. Fortunately it would appear that blood invasion does not take place...."[1,2] His observation was further "corroborated" by pathologic descriptions of "atypical melanocytes" existing within 5 cm of

primary tumors.[1] Unbeknownst to many, Handley had never treated a single melanoma patient himself, but made this assertion based on 1 autopsy.[2] Nonetheless, this concept become the defining dogma.

Alexander Breslow challenged that dogma, demonstrating in 1970 that melanoma thickness correlated most closely with prognosis. He noted that in melanomas less than 0.76 mm, no recurrences or metastases were observed, and thus considered the 5-cm margin to be excessive for thin tumors.[2] In the following decades, uncertainty persisted regarding optimal surgical margins, and treatment varied between "narrow" (2 to 3 cm) and the "standard" 5-cm radical margin.[1,2] This led to the use of narrower surgical margins in the treatment of thinner melanomas with low recurrence rates. In the following decades, uncertainty persisted regarding optimal surgical margins, and treatment varied between "narrow" (2 to 3 cm) and the "standard" 5-cm radical margin. Between 1980 and 2004, 6 landmark RCTs were performed to evaluate the influence of surgical margin width on melanoma recurrence and survival.[1] These 6 RCTs laid the framework upon which the National Comprehensive Cancer Network (NCCN) and American Academy of Dermatology (AAD) established their guidelines recommendations.[3,4] Critically, however, in a meta-analysis of the 6 landmark melanoma RCTs, there was no difference in overall survival or recurrence-free survival between groups treated with narrow or wide surgical margins,[1,5] indicating that tumor thickness and width of clinical surgical margins are not directly correlative. Notably, most melanomas included in these landmark trials were located on the trunk and proximal extremities, leading to a paucity of data for melanomas of the head and neck as well as other special sites.[1]

The advent of MMS, developed and pioneered by Dr Frederic E. Mohs, a general surgeon in the 1930s, revolutionized the definitive management of cutaneous malignancies.[5–7] Unlike traditional WLE, which undergoes standard pathologic grossing and processing using "breadloaf," also known as vertical sectioning and which allows for the histopathologic evaluation of less than 1% of the true surgical margin,[6–9] the Mohs micrographic technique processed fresh-frozen tissue in a method that allowed for complete circumferential peripheral and deep margin assessment in real time, allowing for 100% true surgical margin assessment.[5–7,9–12] This led to tremendous improvements in tumor cure rates and decreased local recurrence and regional nodal disease for cutaneous carcinoma by orders of magnitude.[7,9] Historically, MMS for cutaneous melanomas had been approached with hesitancy and reluctance by many surgeons, given the perceived difficulties in the identification of tumoral melanocytes on fresh-frozen tissue stained with hematoxylin and eosin (H&E); however, with the recent advancements in high-quality, reliable immunohistochemical stains for melanocytes on fresh-frozen tissue, MMS for cutaneous melanoma has been reapproached with great renewed enthusiasm, as it has been shown to provide superior, durable tumor cure rates that are 5 to 20 times better than that achieved with traditional WLE.[5,6,10–24] More recently, it has even been demonstrated that patients who undergo MMS for melanomas may have improved survival over those who undergo traditional WLE[20–24] (**Figs. 1** and **2**).

## Cutaneous Melanomas of the Head and Neck

### General principles

The head and neck, hands, feet, genitalia, and pretibial leg are known to be specialty sites for melanoma. Melanomas of the head and neck make up a considerable proportion of diagnoses at 15.5% to 20.2% of all melanomas.[6,10,11,14,16,25,26] Melanomas of the head and neck have distinct risk factors and associations compared with melanomas of the trunk and proximal extremities. Head and neck melanomas are strongly correlated with chronic sun damage and are diagnosed more commonly in older populations than melanomas on the trunk and proximal extremities; as a result of chronic sun damage, melanomas of the head and neck tend to demonstrate extensive subclinical extent far beyond the clinical boundaries of the tumor.[6,10–12,14,20,21,23,25–30] Melanomas in chronically sun-damaged skin bear a greater mutational burden as well.[14,31] Superficial spreading melanomas and lentigo maligna melanomas make up most melanoma subtypes diagnosed on the head and neck.[6,10,11,14,16,20,21,23,25,26] Head and neck melanomas have a higher risk of disease recurrence and death in comparison with melanomas of the trunk and extremities, with significantly worse overall and disease-free survival even when adjusting for other prognostic factors, including age, Breslow depth, and presence of ulceration.[6,10,11,14,20,21,23,25–27]

### Challenges associated with wide local excision for melanomas on the head and neck

The risk of positive margins, local recurrence, upstaging, and complex reconstruction with flap or graft is higher in melanomas on special anatomic sites in comparison to melanomas of the trunk and proximal extremities.[10,11,14–16,20,21,23,25,32–34] The AAD guidelines on the surgical treatment of melanoma from 2019 state that "surgical excision with histologically negative margins is the recommended and first line treatment for primary cutaneous melanoma of any thickness, as well as for melanoma in situ."[35] However, several studies have found that the anatomic location of melanomas on the head and neck as well as other specialty sites is an independent risk factor associated with greater odds for positive or equivocal margins, because of both the cosmetic and the functional sensitivities of these areas, often putting surgeons at higher risk of noncompliance with recommended traditional clinical surgical margins, as well as extensive subclinical extension beyond the visible tumor boundary, which is notorious for melanomas on the head and neck and those in chronically sun-damaged skin.[10,11,14,16,17,22–24,33,36,37] As a result, in published studies looking at outcomes of melanomas that underwent standard WLE, the average rate of residual positive margins for specialty site melanomas was 9.1%, compared with 1.7% for melanomas on the trunk and extremities,[10,11,14,16,17,22–24,33,36–38] with resultant published local recurrence rates as high as 28% (range, 3%–28%) for melanomas of the head and neck undergoing standard excision versus 3% (range, 1%–3%) for melanomas on the trunk and extremities.[10,11,14,16,17,22–24,33,36–38] Several recently published large-scale prospectively collected studies on melanoma outcomes treated with MMS have illustrated the consequences of extensive subclinical spread of tumors arising on the head and neck, demonstrating that the average clinical margins needed to achieve histologic tumor clearance in 97% of cases is at least 12 mm on the head and neck, versus at least 10 mm for tumors on the trunk and extremities[6,10,11,14,16,22–24,28–30,33] (**Fig. 3**). In melanomas that underwent excision with less than 0.7 cm clinical margins, residual tumor was identified in more than 20% of cases.[11,28,29]

Prevention of local recurrence is a key pillar in the surgical treatment of melanoma, akin to achieving histologically negative margins. In a recently published study evaluating the invasive growth patterns of residual or recurrent melanomas, it was found that 22.6% to 33% of recurrent melanoma in situ cases present with new invasion at a mean Breslow depth 0.94 mm, and 33% of recurrent invasive melanomas of the head and neck demonstrate deeper invasion, with a mean change in Breslow depth from a mean of 1.53 mm to 2.83 mm.[10] Moreover, recurrent melanomas are known to have worse prognoses than primary tumors, even when controlling for Breslow depth and stage.[10,26,27,33,34,39] Because

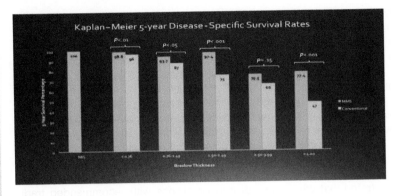

**Fig. 1.** Five-year Kaplan-Meier melanoma-specific survival rates after MMS (n = 1376) compared with published historical controls (n = 15,798), stratified by Breslow depth/T stage. (*From* Valentín-Nogueras SM, Brodland DG, Zitelli JA, et al. Mohs Micrographic Surgery Using MART-1 Immunostain in the Treatment of Invasive Melanoma and Melanoma In Situ. Dermatol Surg. 2016 Jun;42(6):733-44; with permission.)

of both the functional and the cosmetic sensitivities of melanomas arising on the head and neck often resulting in surgeons "cheating the margins" and the well-documented phenomenon of extensive subclinical spread of tumors arising in chronically sun-damaged skin, tumor upstaging during or after definitive treatment is of real concern. This complication is more common in melanomas on specialty sites, particularly in those arising on the head and neck, where approximately 11% of melanoma excision specimens are upstaged, compared with approximately 2% of those arising on the trunk and proximal extremities.[14] If residual melanoma of a higher T stage is discovered in the specimen from WLE, the melanoma may be upstaged. This can alter prognosis and recommendations for additional staging procedures, such as sentinel lymph node biopsy (SLNB), which is further complicated by disruption of draining lymphatics if repair or reconstruction, especially with flap or graft, has already taken place. The need for complex reconstruction with a flap or a graft on a specialty site is much greater than on

the trunk and proximal extremities, 53.7% compared with 10.1%.[15] This need is likely higher because of the need to preserve anatomy and function on these intricate and sensitive anatomic sites. Published NCCN guidelines on the treatment of basal cell carcinoma, squamous cell carcinoma, Merkel cell carcinoma, and dermatofibrosarcoma protuberans recommend holding off on tissue rearranging reconstruction until a tumor is determined to have been cleared based on histologic examination. However, this recommendation is not included in guidelines on the treatment of melanoma despite the increased risk of complications, including recurrence and positive margins especially prevalent in specialty site melanomas.[14]

## Mohs Micrographic Surgery for Cutaneous Melanomas of the Head and Neck

Ensuring comprehensive margin control and histologic clearance of tumor is paramount in optimizing outcomes for patients with melanomas of the head and neck. Given the unique ability of

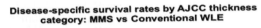

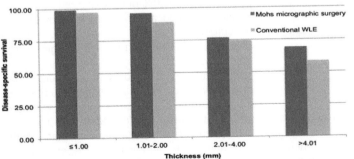

| Tumor thickness | Mohs Micrographic Surgery (95%CI) | Conventional WLE (95%CI) |
|---|---|---|
| ≤1 mm | 99.2(98.5–99.8) | 97.1(96.9–97.4) |
| >1.01 and ≤2 mm | 96.2(93.5–99.0) | 89.1(88.2–89.9) |
| >2.01 and ≤4 mm | 76.6(66.6–88.1) | 74.4(72.8–76.0) |
| >4 mm | 68.8(55.3–85.6) | 58.1(55.5–60.5) |

**Fig. 2.** Five-year Kaplan-Meier melanoma-specific survival rates for invasive melanoma of the trunk and proximal portion of an extremity treated with MMS (N = 1416) compared with historical control values (n = 9129) treated with WLE. AJCC, American Joint Committee on Cancer; CI, confidence interval. (*From* Burnett ME, Brodland DG, Zitelli JA. Long-term outcomes of Mohs micrographic surgery for invasive melanoma of the trunk and proximal portion of the extremities. J Am Acad Dermatol. 2021 Mar;84(3):661-668; with permission.)

## Aggregate analysis

| % Melanoma cleared | Margin (mm) |
|---|---|
| 82% | ≤6 |
| 94-97% | ≤9 |
| 97-99% | ≤12 |

| Location | Margin (mm) |
|---|---|
| To clear 97% tumors on **trunk** | ≤9 |
| To clear 98% tumors on **hands and feet** | ≤12 |
| To clear 97% tumors on **head and neck** | ≤15 |

**Fig. 3.** Clearance rates associated with clinical surgical margins needed to achieve histologic tumor clearance of melanomas based on anatomic location. Residual tumor identified in 21% of cases using 6-mm clinical margins. (*Adapted from* Kunishige JH, Doan L, Brodland DG, Zitelli JA. Comparison of surgical margins for lentigo maligna versus melanoma in situ. J Am Acad Dermatol. 2019 Jul;81(1):204-212; with permission.)

the Mohs technique to provide comprehensive circumferential peripheral and deep margin evaluation with 100% assessment of the true surgical margin, it would be only logical to assume that Mohs surgery confers an intrinsic superiority to standard WLE for tumor margin control. However, this recognition of its superiority was not always met with widespread enthusiasm nor understanding in the early days. Although MMS for melanoma was used by Dr Mohs and several other pioneering surgeons since its inception in the 1950s, the technique was slow to be accepted by all, because of perceived difficulties in interpreting melanocytes on fresh-frozen tissue stained with routine H&E.[40–43] The real revolution in its utilization came into fruition with the development of reliable high-quality immunohistochemical stains used of fresh-frozen tissue in the 1990s.[40–43] This allowed the Mohs surgeon to see melanocytes with much greater precision and clarity, and high-quality stains allowed for greater reliability and consistency in slide quality from case to case. As such, over the course of the last 2 decades, and more recently in the past few years, several landmark large-scale studies have been published demonstrating the superiority of MMS aided with real-time intraoperative immunohistochemical stains in the treatment of cutaneous melanomas: incredibly, long-term, reproducible local tumor cure rates

exceeding 99% at 5 and 10 years have been published in several recent landmark large-scale studies, demonstrating superior tumor cure rates that are 5 to 20 times better than that achieved with traditional WLE.[5,6,10–24,40–43] Moreover, it has been recently demonstrated that patients who undergo MMS for melanomas of the head and neck may have improved overall and disease-specific survival over those who undergo traditional WLE[20–24] (see **Figs. 1** and **2**). Conceptually, superiority in tumor cure rates in the Mohs technique's ability to assess 100% of the margin. As such, the "hard and fast rules" of melanoma excision using arbitrary clinical margins are no longer relevant, as the margin is assessed comprehensively, and in real time, during the time of surgery. As such, comprehensive margin control can be confidently achieved, and this allowed for not only greater histologically confirmed tumor cure rates but also for tissue conservation, if feasible.

### Technique

Although there are several minor variations among surgeons in the specifics of the technique used when performing MMS for melanoma, the general process is summarized as in **Fig. 4**.

Preoperatively, any clinical residual tumor is identified and marked. An initial clinical margin around the tumor, generally consisting of 1 to 3 mm, is identified and marked to be used as a central debulk and positive vertical control. This central debulk is used for final Breslow depth and pathologic staging. Notably, the ability to detect upstaging before reconstruction is also another great advantage of MMS over standard WLE for melanoma: if residual melanoma of a higher T stage is discovered, this can alter prognosis and change management, such as facilitating the need for further prognostication in the form of SLNB. The incidence of postoperative upstaging is nearly 4 times higher in melanomas on the head and neck, where on average 11% of melanomas are upstaged after surgery, compared with 3% on the trunk and proximal extremities.[14] This consequence of postoperative upstaging is further complicated by disruption of draining lymphatics if reconstruction is performed before final Breslow depth and staging, as complex reconstruction involving flaps or grafts may alter the draining lymphatics and affect the results of the SLNB. The need for complex reconstruction with a flap or a graft is much greater for melanomas arising on the head and neck than on the trunk and proximal extremities, averaging approximately 54% compared with 10%.[15] This is due to the inherent need to preserve functional

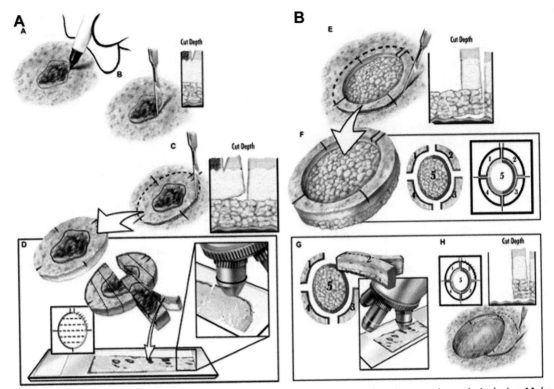

**Fig. 4.** Tissue processing techniques to optimize tumor staging and comprehensive margin analysis during Mohs micrographic surgery for cutaneous melanoma. (*From* Etzkorn JR, Sobanko JF, Elenitsas R, et al. Low recurrence rates for in situ and invasive melanomas using Mohs micrographic surgery with melanoma antigen recognized by T cells 1 (MART-1) immunostaining: tissue processing methodology to optimize pathologic staging and margin assessment. J Am Acad Dermatol. 2015 May;72(5):840 to 50; with permission.)

anatomy and cosmesis in these intricate and sensitive sites. Moreover, MMS has demonstrated even greater sensitivity in detecting occult upstaging that was missed on routine standard pathologic staging, with unanticipated upstaging occurring in nearly 6% of Mohs surgery cases.[44]

After the central debulking is performed, a clinical margin of 3 mm is then used for the initial Mohs layer, which is incised through the subcutis and underneath the depth of the central debulking. This first Mohs layer is processed as fresh-frozen tissue and sectioned in Mohs fashion, then stained with both H&E as well as melanocyte-specific immunohistochemical stain, such as MART-1.[6] Positive margins are defined in congruence to the well-established published parameters defining melanoma histopathology. If any positive margin is identified, a targeted excision of that margin section is performed again, with an additional clinical margin of 2 to 3 mm of normal-appearing skin. This process is repeated until all margins are confirmed tumor free.[6]

Using this intricate technique, superior tumor control is readily achieved and has been demonstrated in several landmark studies, with durable, long-term published cure rates exceeding 99% at 5 and 10 years and local recurrence rates averaging 0.2% to 0.49% published in the literature, compared with local recurrence rates of 5% to 28% with standard WLE demonstrated in historical published controls.[5,6,10–24,40–43]

## SUMMARY

MMS is a highly effective treatment option for cutaneous melanomas of the head and neck. It provides complete margin analysis and is associated with local recurrence rates and equivalent to better melanoma-specific survival rates compared with traditional WLE, even when stratified by Breslow depth. In addition, it allows for tissue conservation, when applicable, and same-day reconstruction of the site. The utilization of MMS should be approached thoughtfully and diligently, as the technique is complex and requires an experienced laboratory team: experience is key and close collaboration with dermatopathologists is key.

## CLINICS CARE POINTS

- Inform patients of the greater risk of recurrence, upstaging, and need for complex reconstruction associated with melanomas of the head and neck.
- Understand that a patient's greatest concern in the treatment of melanoma is ensuring complete tumor removal.
- Mohs micrographic surgery allows for complete tumor removal, confirmation of negative margins, and complete reconstruction on the same day.
- When treating melanomas of the head and neck, remember that these tumors often demonstrate subclinical asymmetric spread and require larger margins for acceptable clearance than melanomas of the trunk and extremities.
- As melanomas of the head and neck present higher risk of upstaging and need for SLNB, when unable to confirm histologically negative margins intraoperatively, as with Mohs surgery, it is prudent to consider delaying tissue rearranging construction until negative margins can be confirmed so as to not disturb the underlying lymphatics.
- When referring for Mohs surgery, referral to a Mohs surgeon who is trained in the intraoperative recognition of melanoma with the use of immunohistochemical staining techniques is essential.

## DISCLOSURE

The authors have no financial disclosures or conflicts of interest to report.

## REFERENCES

1. Angeles CV, Wong SL, Karakousis G. The landmark series: randomized trials examining surgical margins for cutaneous melanoma. Ann Surg Oncol 2020;27(1):3–12.
2. Weyers W. Personalized excision of malignant melanoma-need for a paradigm shift in the beginning era of personalized medicine. Am J Dermatopathol 2019;41:884–96.
3. Ad Hoc Task Force, Connolly SM, Baker DR, et al. AAD/ACMS/ASDSA/ASMS 2012 appropriate use criteria for Mohs micrographic surgery: a report of the American Academy of Dermatology, American College of Mohs Surgery, American Society for Dermatologic Surgery Association, and the American Society for Mohs Surgery. J Am Acad Dermatol 2012;67(4):531–50. Erratum in: J Am Acad Dermatol. 2015 Apr;72(4):748.
4. [Guideline] National Comprehensive Cancer Network. NCCN clinical practice guidelines in oncology: melanoma. NCCN. Available at. http://www.nccn.org/professionals/physician_gls/pdf/melanoma.pdf. [Accessed 31 January 2020]. Version 1.2020 — December 19, 2019.
5. Soleymani T. Understanding margins in the management of cutaneous melanoma. The time for a paradigm shift is now. Dermatol Surg 2021;47(6):827–8.
6. Ellison PM, Zitelli JA, Brodland DG. Mohs micrographic surgery for melanoma: a prospective multicenter study. J Am Acad Dermatol 2019;81(3):767–74.
7. Mansouri B, Bicknell LM, Hill D, et al. Mohs micrographic surgery for the management of cutaneous malignancies. Facial Plast Surg Clin North Am 2017;25(3):291–301.
8. Kimyai-Asadi A, Katz T, Goldberg LH, et al. Margin involvement after the excision of melanoma in situ: the need for complete en face examination of the surgical margins. Dermatol Surg 2007;33(12):1434–9. discussion 1439-41.
9. Chang AE, Ganz PA, Hayes DF, et al. Oncology: an evidence-based approach. 1st ed. Berlin: Springer; 2006.
10. DeBloom JR 2nd, Zitelli JA, Brodland DG. The invasive growth potential of residual melanoma and melanoma in situ. Dermatol Surg 2010;36(8):1251–7.
11. Kunishige JH, Doan L, Brodland DG, et al. Comparison of surgical margins for lentigo maligna versus melanoma in situ. J Am Acad Dermatol 2019;81(1):204–12.
12. Shin TM, Nugent S, Aizman L, et al. Mohs micrographic surgery with MART-1 immunostaining has durable low local recurrence rates for in situ and invasive melanomas. J Am Acad Dermatol 2021;84(1):196–8.
13. Lee MP, Sobanko JF, Shin TM, et al. Evolution of excisional surgery practices for melanoma in the United States. JAMA Dermatol 2019;155(11):1244–51.
14. Rzepecki AK, Hwang CD, Etzkorn JR, et al. The "Rule of 10s" versus the "Rule of 2s": high complication rates after conventional excision with postoperative margin assessment of specialty site versus trunk and proximal extremity melanomas. J Am Acad Dermatol 2021;85(2):442–52.
15. Etzkorn JR, Sobanko JF, Shin TM, et al. Correlation between appropriate use criteria and the frequency of subclinical spread or reconstruction with a flap or graft for melanomas treated with Mohs surgery with

melanoma antigen recognized by T cells 1 immuno-staining. Dermatol Surg 2016;42(4):471–6.

16. Shin TM, Shaikh WR, Etzkorn JR, et al. Clinical and pathologic factors associated with subclinical spread of invasive melanoma. J Am Acad Dermatol 2017;76(4):714–21.

17. Etzkorn JR, Sobanko JF, Elenitsas R, et al. Low recurrence rates for in situ and invasive melanomas using Mohs micrographic surgery with melanoma antigen recognized by T cells 1 (MART-1) immuno-staining: tissue processing methodology to optimize pathologic staging and margin assessment. J Am Acad Dermatol 2015;72(5):840–50. Erratum in: J Am Acad Dermatol. 2017 Nov 17.

18. Etzkorn JR, Tuttle SD, Lim I, et al. Patients prioritize local recurrence risk over other attributes for surgical treatment of facial melanomas-results of a stated preference survey and choice-based conjoint analysis. J Am Acad Dermatol 2018;79(2):210–9.e3.

19. Miller CJ, Giordano CN, Higgins HW 2nd. Mohs micrographic surgery for melanoma: as use increases, so does the need for best practices. JAMA Dermatol 2019;155(11):1225–6.

20. Hanson J, Demer A, Liszewski W, et al. Improved overall survival of melanoma of the head and neck treated with Mohs micrographic surgery versus wide local excision. J Am Acad Dermatol 2020; 82(1):149–55.

21. Cheraghlou S, Christensen SR, Agogo GO, et al. Comparison of survival after Mohs micrographic surgery vs wide margin excision for early-stage invasive melanoma. JAMA Dermatol 2019;155(11): 1252–9.

22. Stigall LE, Brodland DG, Zitelli JA. The use of Mohs micrographic surgery (MMS) for melanoma in situ (MIS) of the trunk and proximal extremities. J Am Acad Dermatol 2016;75(5):1015–21.

23. Valentín-Nogueras SM, Brodland DG, Zitelli JA, et al. Mohs micrographic surgery using MART-1 immunostain in the treatment of invasive melanoma and melanoma in situ. Dermatol Surg 2016;42(6): 733–44.

24. Burnett ME, Brodland DG, Zitelli JA. Long-term outcomes of Mohs micrographic surgery for invasive melanoma of the trunk and proximal portion of the extremities. J Am Acad Dermatol 2021;84(3):661–8.

25. Golger A, Young DS, Ghazarian D, et al. Epidemiological features and prognostic factors of cutaneous head and neck melanoma: a population-based study. Arch Otolaryngol Head Neck Surg 2007; 133(5):442–7.

26. Fadaki N, Li R, Parrett B, et al. Is head and neck melanoma different from trunk and extremity melanomas with respect to sentinel lymph node status and clinical outcome? Ann Surg Oncol 2013;20(9): 3089–97.

27. Lachiewicz AM, Berwick M, Wiggins CL, et al. Survival differences between patients with scalp or neck melanoma and those with melanoma of other sites in the Surveillance, Epidemiology, and End Results (SEER) program. Arch Dermatol 2008;144(4): 515–21.

28. Kunishige JH, Doan L, Brodland DG, et al. 9-mm surgical margin required for both LM and MIS as diagnosed in real-world community practice. J Am Acad Dermatol 2019;81(4):e117–8.

29. Kunishige JH, Brodland DG, Zitelli JA. Margins for standard excision of melanoma in situ. J Am Acad Dermatol 2013;69(1):164.

30. Valentín SM, Brodland DG, Zitelli JA. Optimal treatment for lentigo maligna. Plast Reconstr Surg 2012;130(6):888e–9e.

31. Sanna A, Harbst K, Johansson I, et al. Tumor genetic heterogeneity analysis of chronic sun-damaged melanoma. Pigment Cell Melanoma Res 2020; 33(3):480–9. Erratum in: Pigment Cell Melanoma Res. 2021 Jan;34(1):144.

32. Etzkorn JR, Sharkey JM, Grunyk JW, et al. Frequency of and risk factors for tumor upstaging after wide local excision of primary cutaneous melanoma. J Am Acad Dermatol 2017;77(2):341–8.

33. Miller CJ, Shin TM, Sobanko JF, et al. Risk factors for positive or equivocal margins after wide local excision of 1345 cutaneous melanomas. J Am Acad Dermatol 2017;77(2):333–40.e1.

34. Moehrle M, Kraemer A, Schippert W, et al. Clinical risk factors and prognostic significance of local recurrence in cutaneous melanoma. Br J Dermatol 2004;151(2):397–406.

35. Swetter SM, Tsao H, Bichakjian CK, et al. Guidelines of care for the management of primary cutaneous melanoma. J Am Acad Dermatol 2019; 80(1):208–50.

36. Erickson JL, Velasco JM, Hieken TJ. Compliance with melanoma treatment guidelines in a community teaching hospital: time trends and other variables. Ann Surg Oncol 2008;15(4):1211–7.

37. Blakely AM, Comissiong DS, Vezeridis MP, et al. Suboptimal compliance with National Comprehensive Cancer Network melanoma guidelines: who is at risk? Am J Clin Oncol 2018;41(8):754–9.

38. Möller MG, Pappas-Politis E, Zager JS, et al. Surgical management of melanoma-in-situ using a staged marginal and central excision technique. Ann Surg Oncol 2009;16(6):1526–36.

39. Swetter SM, Thompson JA, Albertini MR, et al. NCCN Guidelines® insights: melanoma: cutaneous, version 2.2021. J Natl Compr Canc Netw 2021; 19(4):364–76.

40. Zitelli JA, Mohs FE, Larson P, et al. Mohs micrographic surgery for melanoma. Dermatol Clin 1989;7(4):833–43.

41. Zitelli JA, Moy RL, Abell E. The reliability of frozen sections in the evaluation of surgical margins for melanoma. J Am Acad Dermatol 1991;24(1):102–6.

42. Griego RD, Zitelli JA. Mohs micrographic surgery using HMB-45 for a recurrent acral melanoma. Dermatol Surg 1998;24(9):1003–6.

43. Bricca GM, Brodland DG, Zitelli JA. Immunostaining melanoma frozen sections: the 1-hour protocol. Dermatol Surg 2004;30(3):403–8.

44. Cherpelis BS, Moore R, Ladd S, et al. Comparison of MART-1 frozen sections to permanent sections using a rapid 19-minute protocol. Dermatol Surg 2009; 35(2):207–13.

# Management of Regional Lymph Nodes in Head and Neck Melanoma

Mica D.E. Glaun, MD[a,b], Zipei Feng, MD, PhD[a,b], Miriam Lango, MD[b,*]

## KEYWORDS

- Head and neck cutaneous melanoma • Sentinel node biopsy • Completion neck dissection
- Adjuvant melanoma treatment

## KEY POINTS

- Tumor thickness and ulceration remain the most powerful predictors of melanoma-specific survival.
- Sentinel lymph node biopsy is indicated for T1b and greater as well as T1a with adverse features.
- Completion lymph node dissection for patients with positive sentinel lymph nodes should be considered; surgery improves disease-free, but not disease-specific, survival. Active surveillance with ultrasound may be an acceptable alternative. Consultation with oncology for systemic therapy is indicated.
- The role of radiation therapy, shown to decrease nodal field relapse but not improve overall survival, continues to evolve.
- The use of immune checkpoint inhibitors and targeted therapies inhibiting oncogenic signaling proteins have improved the survival of patients with advanced stage disease.

## INTRODUCTION

In 1898, surgical oncologist Dr Herbert Snow wrote, "it is essential to remove, whenever possible, those lymph glands which first receive the infective protoplasm, and bar its entrance into the blood, before they have undergone increase in bulk... It was, and unfortunately, too often still is, the custom to neglect the infected glands unless palpably enlarged."[1] Investigation into the management of locoregional lymph nodes for melanoma treatment continued onward from this point, producing large bodies of data driving a flourishing section of evidence-based surgical oncology. The head and neck region is the second most common site for melanoma, representing 20% to 30% of all melanomas.[2,3] Disease-specific outcomes for melanoma of the head and neck remains debated within the literature with some studies suggesting worse prognosis due to subsite and others solely identifying ulceration and tumor thickness as the factors portending worse outcomes.[2] Multidisciplinary research continues to enrich clinicians' understanding of the most appropriate treatment of primary melanoma and its nodal basin. A focus on the treatment of regional lymph nodes from head and neck melanoma is provided herein.

## RISK FACTORS FOR LYMPH NODE METASTASES IN HEAD AND NECK MELANOMA

Melanoma is the most aggressive form of skin cancer, noted to be the fourth most common cancer in men and fifth most common cancer in women. At present, the incidence of melanoma is increasing faster than any other cancer in men and faster than any cancer other than lung cancer in women. That said, the mortality rate of melanoma remains

[a] Department of Otolaryngology, Baylor College of Medicine, 1977 Butler Boulevard, Suite E5.200, Houston, TX 77030, USA; [b] Department of Head and Neck Surgery, MD Anderson Cancer Center, 1515 Holcombe Boulevard, Houston, TX 77030, USA
* Corresponding author.
E-mail address: MNLango@mdanderson.org

Oral Maxillofacial Surg Clin N Am 34 (2022) 273–281
https://doi.org/10.1016/j.coms.2021.11.001
1042-3699/22/© 2021 Elsevier Inc. All rights reserved.

less than 5%.[2,4] Risk factors for melanoma include genetic predisposition, age greater than 60 years, multiple blistering sunburns, fair skin, multiple atypical nevi, other nonmelanoma skin cancers, immunosuppression, and childhood malignancy. In recent years, young adults, particularly women between the ages of 25 and 39 years have had an increased incidence of melanoma likely due to increase popularity of both outdoor and indoor tanning. Lastly, varying medications have been linked to melanoma in a few cases without direct causality yet confirmed.[4–6]

The most widely accepted risk factors for lymph node metastases include primary tumor thickness and ulceration, which are reflected in melanoma staging. The eighth edition of melanoma staging from the American Joint Committee of Cancer was published in 2017 after the analysis of more than 43,000 patients identified from 10 international centers identifying factors affecting melanoma-specific survival (MSS). Thickness remains the single most powerful predictor of MSS and thus guides T staging. Tumor ulceration has been found to double local recurrence, double regional recurrence, and reduce survival rate by 20% to 30%, thus further differentiating T staging.[7] Although within the latest American Joint Committee on Cancer staging mitotic rate has been removed from staging, it is also a predictor of MSS and can aid clinicians in deciding whether or not to pursue sentinel lymph node (SLN) biopsy in thinner melanomas.

## SENTINEL LYMPH NODE BIOPSY FOR HEAD AND NECK MELANOMA

The concept of SLNs was first described by Rudolf Virchow in patients with tattoos. The SLN was the first lymph node to capture pigment deposits from the skin and identify the lymph node at greatest risk of harboring occult metastases from a primary tumor. Because only a handful of lymph nodes are sampled, the procedure is considered minimally invasive. SLN mapping identifies a small number of lymph nodes among high numbers at risk. The first paper published on SLN biopsy was by surgical oncologist Dr Donald Morton and dermatopathologist Dr Alistair Cochran in 1992. Their proposal for SLN biopsy for early stage melanoma was credited as producing a resurgence of modern medicine toward SLN biopsy.[8]

SLN biopsy served as the basis for several Multicenter Selective Lymphadenectomy Trials (MSLTs). MSLT-1 was made up of 1661 randomized patients with a 10-year follow-up.[9–12] The study randomized patients into a wide local excision and nodal observation group and a wide local with SLN biopsy group. Within the sentinel node group, if the node was positive, completion lymph node dissection (CLND) was performed. If the SLN was negative, the patient was observed, and if nodal recurrence occurred, CLND was then performed. In the wide local and observation group, CLND was performed only if nodal recurrence was found via surveillance imaging. The primary endpoint studied within the MSLT-1 was MSS at 10-year follow-up. The secondary endpoints were disease-free survival, survival without tumor ± SLN dissection (SLND), and incidence of SLND positivity.

MSLT-1 validated SLN biopsy as a minimally invasive diagnostic and staging intervention for intermediate-thickness melanomas without clinical evidence of nodal metastases. The 10-year MSS rate was 62.1 ± 4.8% among patients with metastasis identified by SLN biopsy versus 85.1 ± 1.5% for those without metastasis, increasing the risk of death more than 3-fold. The status of the sentinel node was the strongest prognostic factor for disease-free survival and overall prognosis. The frequency of nodal metastasis in an SLN was 20.8%. Patients with melanomas of the head and neck were not subject to greater rates of recurrence of melanoma-specific death.[9]

Nevertheless, the identification of metastases with SLN biopsy followed by completion lymphadenectomy did not improve MSS relative to observation alone, although lymphadenectomy resulted in lower rates of recurrence and improved disease-free survival. A subset analysis of the trial suggested early completion lymphadenectomy could result in improvements in survival, but 2 subsequent trials that tested this hypothesis found no effect.[13,14] Completion lymphadenectomy identified additional positive non-SLNs in 12% to 24%. However, the presence of positive non-SLNs has been associated with high rates of distant metastases; for this reason, patients may be less likely to benefit from completion lymphadenectomy despite high rates of occult disease.[15] The number of clinically occult lymph node metastases have been incorporated into melanoma staging.

SLN biopsies in head and neck sites were believed to be less reliable than those from other sites due to variability in drainage pathways in the head and neck. The accuracy of SLN biopsy has been studied in head and neck melanomas specifically. A study from the University of Michigan addressed the accuracy of SLN biopsy specifically for head and neck melanoma.[16] Within this study, 353 patients were recruited with a mean follow-up of 35 months. Nineteen percent of patients were found to have one positive SLN and all but one of these patients went on to have a

CLND. One-quarter of the patients in the CLND group had at least 1 positive non-SLN. The study's false-omission rate was 4.2%. Stated differently, their data suggest that only 4.2% of patients will recur in any regional basin after a negative SLN biopsy in the head and neck.[16] Consequently, SLN biopsy for intermediate-depth melanoma represents the standard of care and is most accurate when performed at the time of the primary melanoma excision.

To summarize current recommendations in regard to SLN biopsy

- Perform SLN biopsy for:
  o T1b and greater
  o T1a with other adverse features including mitotic index of 2 or greater, lymphovascular invasion
    - T1a without adverse features has less than a 5% chance of finding a diseased SLN
  o May also be considered for: isolated in-transit metastases or local recurrence of a primary melanoma without clinically or radiographically evident regional or distant metastases
  o Intraoperatively excise in-transit sentinel nodes and remove any nodes with greater than 10% of the highest sentinel node's gamma count
- Tumor thickness is the most reliable predictor of a positive SLN
- For clinical stage 1 to 2, SLN pathologic status is the strongest predictor of survival; positive SLNs are considered an indication for adjuvant therapies

## NECK DISSECTION FOR HEAD AND NECK MELANOMA

Lymphadenectomy in the head and neck consists of planned neck dissection for clinically evident nodal disease or completion neck dissection for positive SLNs. According to current guidelines, melanomas presenting with nodal, but not distant, metastases should undergo primary excision and neck dissection and/or parotidectomy followed by adjuvant systemic therapies such as nivolumab, pembrolizumab, or dabrafenib and trametinib for BRAF V600E-mutated melanomas. Patients with bulky nodal disease at high risk for recurrence or those with unresectable disease should be considered for neoadjuvant systemic therapy, preferably on clinical trial, after multidisciplinary consultation. Adjuvant nodal radiotherapy may be used in select patients with multiple involved lymph nodes and/or extranodal extension to decrease regional recurrences.

Completion neck dissection may be considered after findings of a positive SLN. The proposed benefits of CLND are reducing residual disease in non-sentinel nodes, increasing prognostic value, and enabling patients to enter clinical trials. The negative aspects of performing CLND include cost and morbidity of surgery. As noted previously, CLND has been associated with improvements in disease-free survival, but not melanoma-specific mortality.[13,14] In MSLT-2,[13] CLND conferred higher rates of regional disease control in the CLND group compared with the observation after positive SLN biopsy ($92 \pm 1.0\%$ vs $77 \pm 1.5\%$, $P < .001$).[13] However, representation of primary lesions within the head and neck within the MSLT-2 trial was small. Only 13% or 241 patients had head and neck melanoma, with 113 undergoing CLND. Patients with melanomas arising in head and neck sites were excluded from the DeCOG-SLT study.[14] Thus, findings from these studies may not be generalizable.

The rationale for completion lymphadenectomy for SLN positive head and neck melanomas include the limitations of prior trials and the relatively lesser morbidity of completion rather than salvage surgery in head and neck sites. Furthermore, neck dissection and parotidectomy are rarely associated with significant lymphedema in the absence or radiotherapy. The morbidity of completion surgery for head and neck melanomas must be weighed against the risk of locoregional recurrence.[17] Active surveillance may be considered, including ultrasound of the at-risk lymph node basin every 4 months for the first 2 years and every 6 months for years 3 to 5.[15] Regardless of whether completion surgery or active surveillance is selected, systemic therapy such as nivolumab, pembrolizumab, or dabrafenib and trametinib for BRAF V600E-mutated melanomas should be considered. A survey of National Comprehensive Cancer Network Melanoma Panel members indicated that completion surgery for a positive SLN should not be factored into the decision for adjuvant therapy.[15] Other factors such as the number of metastases, the size and location of deposits, identification of in-transit disease , or primary tumor ulceration play a greater role in decisions to initiate systemic therapy.

## UNKNOWN PRIMARY MELANOMA

Melanoma that presents as either nodal disease or distant metastasis without a known primary is rare. Originally described by Dr Das Gupta, 4 rigorous exclusion criteria need to be met before diagnosing melanoma of unknown primary (MUP).[18] These criteria include (1) evidence of previous skin excision, electrodessication, cauterization, or other surgical manipulation of a mole, freckle, birthmark, paronychia, or skin blemish; (2) evidence of previous orbital exenteration or enucleation; (3) evidence of metastatic melanoma in a draining lymph node with a scar in the area of skin supplying that lymph node basin; and (4) lack of a nonthorough physical examination, including the absence of an ophthalmologic, anal, and genital examination. More than 75% of patients with MUP present with nodal disease with 15% of this cohort composed of cervical lymphadenopathy.[19] Treatment of MUP often involves surgical lymphadenectomy with or without adjuvant chemotherapy, radiation, or immunotherapy. Compared with melanoma with known primary, the survival data for MUP are variable[20–22] with median survival between 24 months and more than 10 years for those with nodal disease only and 3 to 14 months for visceral metastasis.[15,23] Spontaneous regression of skin nevi and metastatic disease has been found in MUP, and gene signature has demonstrated a more proinflammatory state.[24] As a result, the response to checkpoint blockade may be more favorable in this population.[22] Management of MUP is heterogeneous and undergoing evolution due to relative rarity of the disease with current treatment typically including lymphadenectomy with or without adjuvant therapy.

## RADIOTHERAPY USE IN HEAD AND NECK MELANOMA

With the development of targeted and immunotherapy in the last decade, systemic therapy has become the preferred treatment option for metastatic melanoma. The role of radiation therapy, outside of a trial setting, is to improve locoregional control in patients with high-risk features such as desmoplastic melanoma, extranodal spread or matted nodes, multiple lymph nodes, and 3 cm or greater cervical nodes.[25–30] Radiotherapy has also been used in a palliative setting for metastasis that causes significant pain or obstruction. Nodal basin radiation has demonstrated excellent local control after lymph node biopsy compared with formal dissection.[31] No survival benefit from conventional radiotherapy has been demonstrated thus far, however, due to reported high rates of distant metastases.[32]

However, radiation therapy is a rapidly evolving field. We now know that radiation can induce the expression of many immune modulatory molecules such as programmed-death ligand 1 (PD-L1) and potentially cause an immunogenic cell death that results in antigen priming.[33,34] Radiation also causes an influx of macrophages that release molecules such as tumor growth factor beta to dampen the immune response.[35] Combinations of radiotherapy with immunotherapy are being actively investigated to treat recurrent melanomas.[36]

## IMMUNOTHERAPY IN HEAD AND NECK MELANOMA

Over the last decade, it has been increasingly realized that treatment failure results from a deficiency of the immune system to contain and eliminate the cancer. The introduction and advancement of immunotherapy fundamentally changed the way melanoma was treated. These various agents are discussed in the following section.

### Checkpoint Blockade Therapy

The homeostasis of the adaptive immune response is tightly regulated. In order for a T cell to be activated and proliferate, it needs the engagement of antigen to T-cell receptor (TCR) (signal 1), the binding of CD80/86 from antigen-presenting cells to the costimulatory receptor CD28 (signal 2), and a proinflammatory cytokine milieu such as interleukin-12 (IL-12) and IL-2 (signal 3).[37] The proliferation and maturation of these antigen-specific T cells serve as the basis of an antitumor immune response.[38] Checkpoint receptors are negative regulators of this response and act as "brakes" to restore proper homeostasis.[38] They are often hijacked by tumor cells to resist immune-mediated elimination. Blocking immune checkpoints with antibodies subsequently results in restoration of suppressed T-cell function and heightened antitumor T-cell response. Anti-CTLA-4 and Anti-PD-1 has resulted in unprecedented efficacy for the treatment of melanoma.[39,40] Other checkpoint molecules will be briefly reviewed here as well.

CTLA-4 or cytotoxic T lymphocyte–associated protein 4 is a CD28 homologue expressed on the surface of T cells including early activated CD8 T cells and regulatory T cells. Engagement of CTLA-4 results in direct inhibition of TCR signaling and reduction of signal 2 for activation.[41–43] Anti-CTLA-4 antibody was the first checkpoint blockade agent approved for treatment of metastatic melanoma based on a randomized phase III study demonstrating increased survival compared with vaccine alone.[39] Currently, the 10-year overall survival in patients treated with ipilimumab is roughly 20%.[44]

PD-1 is another inhibitory receptor on the surface of activated T cells. Similar to CTLA-4, engagement of anti-PD-1 results in TCR signaling inhibition.[45–47] This process is frequently hijacked by melanoma, which can express high levels of PD-L1, the ligand for PD-1. Disruption of this axis through PD-1 blockade in clinical trials demonstrated significantly improved survival for melanoma compared with conventional agents, which led to the approval for anti-PD-1 in 2014.[48] Similarly, PD-L1 blockade has shown promising results and is currently approved in combination with BRAF inhibitor in advanced BRAF-mutant melanoma.[49]

LAG-3 or lymphocyte-activation gene 3 is another molecule found on the surface of both effector T cells and regulatory T cells that functions to negatively regulate CD8 T-cell activation and growth.[50] Disruption of LAG-3 signaling has shown significant promise. The latest RELATIVITY-047 trial has most recently revealed that anti-LAG-3 met its primary endpoint in progression-free survival.[51]

## Cytokine-Based Therapy

Cytokines are endogenous molecular signals that can modulate immune response in various ways. Many of these have been shown to generate a robust antitumor immune response including IL-2, IL-12, IL-15, IL-21, and interferons.[37] Out of these, IL-2 is perhaps one of the most studied. It is a protein that functions to stimulate T-cell proliferation and differentiation through the IL-2 receptor; this effect is not limited to CD4 and CD8 T cells but also regulatory T cells, which acts as a negative feedback mechanism to prevent immune overactivity.[52,53] Systemic administration of high-dose IL-2 remains a key treatment strategy for treatment of metastatic melanoma. Although limited to patients with good performance status due to toxicity, high-dose IL-2 induces objective clinical response in 15% to 25% of patients with metastatic melanoma with complete response around 10%.[54–57] Importantly, of the patients achieving complete response, vast majority remains disease free for decades.[54]

## Adoptive T-Cell Therapy with Autologous T Cells

Adoptive T-cell therapy involves harvesting T cells from autologous tumor, followed by ex-vivo expansion and tumor-specificity test and reinfusion into a nonmyeloablative lymphodepleted patient.[58,59] High-dose IL-2 is also administered concurrently to support clonal expansion of these transferred T cells. In melanoma, recovery rate of tumor-specific T cells range from 35% to 70% of patients, and objective response rate is 50% to 75%.[60–62] Similar to other types of immunotherapy, the response rate is durable in more than 95% of complete responders.[61] Major limitations of adoptive T-cell therapies include relative high cost and variable recovery rate limiting its generalizability.[63] Certain biomarkers such as ratio of CD8+ to FoxP3+ T cells can help to predict success of culturing these tumor-specific T cells.[63]

## Immune System Agonists

Immune system agonists are costimulatory receptors that can significantly increase T-cell proliferation, differentiation, and overall function.

OX40 is a member of the tumor necrosis factor receptor (TNFR) superfamily. Activation of OX40 through an agonist antibody can increase CD4 and CD8 T cell priming and ultimately effector function.[64–66] Clinically, OX40 agonist has demonstrated to be safe in phase I clinical trials, and current trials in melanoma are underway.[67]

As OX40, 4-1BB is another member of the TNFR superfamily that is on activated T cells and NK cells. Its activation by 4-1BBL or agonist antibody on CD8 and CD4 T cells results in increased proliferation, cytokine production, and survival.[68–70] Trials with 4-1BB agonist seem to be well tolerated and demonstrated promise.[71]

## SUMMARY/DISCUSSION

Treatment of melanoma is steeped in a rich history of large multidisciplinary studies and evidence-based surgical oncology. Sentinel lymph node biopsy was a novel technique which dramatically improved staging and transformed the standard of care. Completion node dissection within the head and neck is easily accessible with relatively low morbidity and thus continues to be recommended with active imaging surveillance accepted as well. Seldomly, patients present with metastatic melanoma of unknown primary site and must undergo a vigorous examination to rule out any primary lesion. Interestingly, one school of thought is that MUP of visceral organs may originate from ectopic melanocytes or melanoblastic cells that occasionally found to be present in lymph nodes or gastrointestinal tract.[72,73] Treatment is similar to those with metastatic melanoma originating from a known primary site, which consists of immunotherapy, surgery, or radiation. Survival is variable, partly secondary to the rarity of the disease itself. There are a handful of historic studies demonstrating favorable prognosis compared with melanoma with known primary; however, more studies are needed especially in the era of immunotherapy.

Perhaps the most important breakthrough in the last decade is the advancement in immunotherapy led by checkpoint blockades. The response rate is unprecedented for systemic treatment of metastatic melanoma;, more importantly, the favorable results tend to be durable. Within a short period of time, immunotherapy has become an integral part of treatment regimens. Currently, most of the attention is focused on PD-1 and CTLA-4 axis treatments as monotherapies or in combination with other modalities such as radiotherapy. Traditionally known to be an important adjunct in locoregional control for the treatment of melanoma of the head and neck, failure of radiotherapy stems from the high likelihood of distant metastatic disease in patients with metastatic lymph nodes. Within the last decade, one of the rapidly growing areas of interest for radiotherapy is its immuno-modulatory effect and utility when used in combination with immunotherapy. Few of these trials have been completed[36] and more are underway.

Lastly, despite significant promise of immunotherapy for the treatment of melanoma, failures do occur not infrequently. Other types of immunotherapy options are available or are in development. As we develop more and more immunotherapeutics, predictive biomarkers become increasingly important. Different from targeted therapies for which mutations can be assessed rapidly and accurately to guide therapy, assessing responses to immunotherapy and developing novel biomarkers have been more challenging. Currently, the only Food and Drug Administration–approved biomarker for checkpoint blockade is PD-L1 status; however, this treatment is problematic, as patients with negative PD-L1 can respond to checkpoint blockade and vice versa.[74] Other methodologies, such as analysis of multiple immune populations and development of signatures have shown promise.[63,75] Going forward, it will be important to consider obtaining wide variety of samples including genomics, proteomic, flow cytometric, and immunohistochemical data for each clinical trial to help understand more about the tumor microenvironment and guide therapy.

## CLINICS CARE POINTS

- Tumor thickness and ulceration are the most powerful predictors of MSS.

- SLN biopsy is strongly recommended for head and neck melanomas staged T1b and greater, as well as some T1a melanomas.
- Completion node dissection for patients with positive SLNs may improve regional recurrence but does not improve MSS; systemic therapy options should be considered.

## DISCLOSURE

No commercial or financial conflicts of interest for any authors.

## REFERENCES

1. Rebecca VW, Sondak VK, Smalley KSM. A brief history of melanoma: from mummies to mutations. Melanoma Res 2012;22(2):114–22.
2. Goepfert RP, Myers JN, Gershenwald JE. Updates in the evidence-based management of cutaneous melanoma. Head Neck 2020;42(11):3396–404.
3. Pathak I, Brien CJO, Petersen-schaeffer K, et al. Do nodal metastases from cutaneous melanoma of the head & neck follow a clinicall predictable pattern? Head Neck 2001;23(9):785–90.
4. Rastrelli M, Tropea S, Rossi CR, et al. Melanoma: epidemiology, risk factors, pathogenesis, diagnosis and classification. In Vivo (Brooklyn) 2014;1012: 1005–11.
5. Ferrucci L, Vogel R, Cartmel B, et al. Indoor tanning in businesses and homes and risk of melanoma and non-melanoma skin cancer in two US case-control studies. J Am Acad Dermatol 2015;71(5):882–7.
6. Nergard-martin j, Caldwell C, Barr M, et al. Perceptions of tanning risk among melanoma patients with a history of indoor tanning. Cutis 2018;101(1). 47;50; 55.
7. Balch BCM, Soong S, Gershenwald JE, et al. Prognostic factors analysis of 17, 600 melanoma patients: melanoma staging system. J Clin Oncol 2001;19(16):3622–34.
8. Morton D, Wen D, Wong J. Technical details of intraoperative lymphatic mapping for early stage melanoma. Arch Surg 1992;127:392–9.
9. Morton D, Thompson J, Cochren A, et al. Sentinel-node biopsy or nodal observation in melanoma. N Engl J Med 2006;355(13):1307–17.
10. Faries M, Wanek L, Elashoff D, et al. Predictors of occult nodal metastasis in patients with thin melanoma. Arch Surg 2010;145(2):137–42.
11. Howard JH, Thompson JF, Mozzillo N, et al. Metastasectomy for distant metastatic melanoma: analysis of data from the first Multicenter Selective Lymphadenectomy Trial (MSLT-I). Ann Surg Oncol 2012; 19(8):2547–55.

12. Morton DL, Thompson JF, Cochran AJ, et al. Final trial report of sentinel-node biopsy versus nodal observation in melanoma. N Engl J Med 2014; 370(7):599–609.

13. Faries M, Thompson J, Cochran R, et al. Completion dissection or observation for sentinel-node metastasis in melanoma. N Engl J Med 2017;376(23): 2211–22.

14. Leiter U, Stadler R, Mauch C, et al. Complete lymph node dissection versus no dissection in patients with sentinel lymph node biopsy positive melanoma (De-COG-SLT): a multicentre, randomised, phase 3 trial. Lancet Oncol 2016;17(6):757–67.

15. National Comprehensive Cancer Network. Melanoma: cutaneous (Version 2.2021). Available at: http://www.nccn.org/professionals/physician_gls/ pdf/cutaneous_melanoma.pdf. [Accessed 7 September 2021].

16. Erman AB, Collar RM, Griffith KA, et al. Sentinel lymph node biopsy is accurate and prognostic in head and neck melanoma. Cancer 2012;118(4): 1040–7.

17. Farlow JL, McLean SA, Peddireddy N, et al. Impact of completion lymphadenectomy on quality of life for head and neck cutaneous melanoma. Otolaryngol Head Neck Surg 2021. 1945998211007442.

18. Das Gupta T, Bowden L, Berg J. Malignant melanoma of unknown primary origin. Surg Gynecol Obstet 1963;117:341–5.

19. Gos A, Jurkowska M, van Akkooi A, et al. Molecular characterization and patient outcome of melanoma nodal metastases and an unknown primary site. Ann Surg Oncol 2014;21(13):4317–23.

20. Lee CC, Faries MB, Wanek LA, et al. Improved survival after lymphadenectomy for nodal metastasis from an unknown primary melanoma. J Clin Oncol 2008;26(4):535–41.

21. Cormier JN, Xing Y, Feng L, et al. Metastatic melanoma to lymph nodes in patients with unknown primary sites. Cancer 2006;106(9):2012–20.

22. Gambichler T, Chatzipantazi M, Schröter U, et al. Patients with melanoma of unknown primary show better outcome under immune checkpoint inhibitor therapy than patients with known primary: preliminary results. Oncoimmunology 2019;8(12): e1677139.

23. Verver D, van der Veldt AAM, van Akkooi ACJ, et al. Treatment of melanoma of unknown primary in the era of immunotherapy and targeted therapy: a Dutch population-based study. Int J Cancer 2020; 146(1):26–34.

24. Haratani K, Hayashi H, Takahama T, et al. Clinical and immune profiling for cancer of unknown primary site. J Immunother Cancer 2019;7(1):251.

25. Henderson MA, Burmeister BH, Ainslie J, et al. Adjuvant lymph-node field radiotherapy versus observation only in patients with melanoma at high risk of further lymph-node field relapse after lymphadenectomy (ANZMTG 01.02/TROG 02.01): 6-year follow-up of a phase 3, randomised controlled trial. Lancet Oncol 2015;16(9):1049–60.

26. O'Brien C, Petersen-Schaefer K, Stevens GN, et al. Adjuvant radiotherapy following neck dissection and parotidectomy for metastatic malignant melanoma. Head Neck 1997;19(7):589–94.

27. Bonnen MD, Ballo MT, Myers JN, et al. Elective radiotherapy provides regional control for patients with cutaneous melanoma of the head and neck. Cancer 2004;100(2):383–9.

28. Ballo MT, Ross MI, Cormier JN, et al. Combined-modality therapy for patients with regional nodal metastases from melanoma. Int J Radiat Oncol Biol Phys 2006;64(1):106–13.

29. Rossi M, Pellegrini C, Cardelli L, et al. Melanoma: diagnostic and management implications. Dermatol Pr Concept 2019;9(1):10–6.

30. Guadagnolo BA, Myers JN, Zagars GK. Role of postoperative irradiation for patients with bilateral cervical nodal metastases from cutaneous melanoma: a critical assessment. Head Neck 2010; 32(6):708–13.

31. Ballo MT, Garden AS, Myers JN, et al. Melanoma metastatic to cervical lymph nodes: can radiotherapy replace formal dissection after local excision of nodal disease? Head Neck 2005;27(8): 718–21.

32. Owens JM, Roberts DB, Myers JN. The role of postoperative adjuvant radiation therapy in the treatment of mucosal melanomas of the head and neck region. Arch Otolaryngol Head Neck Surg 2003;129(8): 864–8.

33. Golden EB, Apetoh L. Radiotherapy and immunogenic cell death. Semin Radiat Oncol 2015;25(1): 11–7.

34. Crittenden MR, Zebertavage L, Kramer G, et al. Tumor cure by radiation therapy and checkpoint inhibitors depends on pre-existing immunity. Sci Rep 2018;8(1):1–15.

35. Young KH, Gough MJ, Crittenden M. Tumor immune remodeling by TGFβ inhibition improves the efficacy of radiation therapy. Oncoimmunology 2015;4(3):1–2.

36. Curti B, Crittenden M, Seung SK, et al. Randomized phase II study of stereotactic body radiotherapy and interleukin-2 versus interleukin-2 in patients with metastatic melanoma. J Immunother Cancer 2020; 8(1):1–10.

37. Parham P. The immune system. 2005th edition. New York (NY): Garland Science; 1950.

38. Pardoll DM. The blockade of immune checkpoints in cancer immunotherapy. Nat Rev Cancer 2012;12(4): 252–64.

39. Hodi FS, O'Day SJ, McDermott DF, et al. Improved survival with ipilimumab in patients with metastatic melanoma. N Engl J Med 2010;363(8):711–23.

40. Wolchok JD, Kluger H, Callahan MK, et al. Nivolumab plus ipilimumab in advanced melanoma. N Engl J Med 2013;369(2):122–33.

41. Guntermann C, Alexander DR. CTLA-4 suppresses proximal TCR signaling in resting human CD4(+) T cells by inhibiting ZAP-70 Tyr(319) phosphorylation: a potential role for tyrosine phosphatases. J Immunol 2002;168(9):4420–9.

42. Hurwitz AA, Yu TF, Leach DR, et al. CTLA-4 blockade synergizes with tumor-derived granulocyte-macrophage colony-stimulating factor for treatment of an experimental mammary carcinoma. Proc Natl Acad Sci U S A 1998;95(17):10067–71.

43. Leach DR, Krummel MF, Allison JP. Enhancement of antitumor immunity by CTLA-4 blockade. Science 1996;271(5256):1734–6.

44. Schadendorf D, Hodi FS, Robert C, et al. Pooled analysis of long-term survival data from phase II and phase III trials of ipilimumab in unresectable or metastatic melanoma. J Clin Oncol 2015;33(17): 1889–94.

45. Agata Y, Kawasaki A, Nishimura H, et al. Expression of the PD-1 antigen on the surface of stimulated mouse T and B lymphocytes. Int Immunol 1996; 8(5):765–72.

46. Freeman GJ, Long AJ, Iwai Y, et al. Engagement of the PD-1 immunoinhibitory receptor by a novel B7 family member leads to negative regulation of lymphocyte activation. J Exp Med 2000;192(7): 1027–34.

47. Akbay EA, Koyama S, Carretero J, et al. Activation of the PD-1 pathway contributes to immune escape in EGFR-driven lung tumors. Cancer Discov 2013; 3(12):1355–63.

48. Robert C, Long GV, Brady B, et al. Nivolumab in previously untreated melanoma without BRAF mutation. N Engl J Med 2015;372(4):320–30.

49. Gutzmer R, Stroyakovskiy D, Gogas H, et al. Atezolizumab, vemurafenib, and cobimetinib as first-line treatment for unresectable advanced BRAF^V600 mutation-positive melanoma (IMspire150): primary analysis of the randomised, double-blind, placebo-controlled, phase 3 trial. Lancet 2020;395(10240):1835–44.

50. Graydon CG, Mohideen S, Fowke KR. LAG3's enigmatic mechanism of action. Front Immunol 2021;11: 3444.

51. Lipson EJ, Tawbi HA-H, Schadendorf D, et al. Relatlimab (RELA) plus nivolumab (NIVO) versus NIVO in first-line advanced melanoma: primary phase III results from RELATIVITY-047 (CA224-047). J Clin Oncol 2021;39(15_suppl):9503.

52. Scheffold A, Huhn J, Hofer T. Regulation of CD4+CD25+ regulatory T cell activity: it takes (IL-) two to tango. Eur J Immunol 2005;35(5):1336–41.

53. Curtsinger JM, Schmidt CS, Mondino A, et al. Inflammatory cytokines provide a third signal for activation of naive CD4+ and CD8+ T cells. J Immunol 1999;162(6):3256–62.

54. Payne R, Glenn L, Hoen H, et al. Durable responses and reversible toxicity of high-dose interleukin-2 treatment of melanoma and renal cancer in a Community Hospital Biotherapy Program. J Immunother Cancer 2014;2:13.

55. Atkins MB, Kunkel L, Sznol M, et al. High-dose recombinant interleukin-2 therapy in patients with metastatic melanoma: long-term survival update. Cancer J Sci Am 2000;6(Suppl 1):S11–4.

56. Barth RJ Jr, Mule JJ, Spiess PJ, et al. Interferon gamma and tumor necrosis factor have a role in tumor regressions mediated by murine CD8+ tumor-infiltrating lymphocytes. J Exp Med 1991;173(3): 647–58.

57. Rosenberg SA, Lotze MT, Muul LM, et al. A progress report on the treatment of 157 patients with advanced cancer using lymphokine-activated killer cells and interleukin-2 or high-dose interleukin-2 alone. N Engl J Med 1987;316(15):889–97.

58. Aebersold P, Hyatt C, Johnson S, et al. Lysis of autologous melanoma cells by tumor-infiltrating lymphocytes: association with clinical response. J Natl Cancer Inst 1991;83(13):932–7.

59. Dudley ME, Wunderlich JR, Shelton TE, et al. Generation of tumor-infiltrating lymphocyte cultures for use in adoptive transfer therapy for melanoma patients. J Immunother 2003;26(4):332–42.

60. Rosenberg SA, Restifo NP, Yang JC, et al. Adoptive cell transfer: a clinical path to effective cancer immunotherapy. Nat Rev Cancer 2008;8(4):299–308.

61. Rosenberg SA, Yang JC, Sherry RM, et al. Durable complete responses in heavily pretreated patients with metastatic melanoma using T-cell transfer immunotherapy. Clin Cancer Res 2011;17(13): 4550–7.

62. Wu R, Forget MA, Chacon J, et al. Adoptive T-cell therapy using autologous tumor-infiltrating lymphocytes for metastatic melanoma: current status and future outlook. Cancer J 2012;18(2):160–75.

63. Feng Z, Puri S, Moudgil T, et al. Multispectral imaging of formalin-fixed tissue predicts ability to generate tumor-infiltrating lymphocytes from melanoma. J Immunother Cancer 2015;3:47.

64. Bell RB, Leidner RS, Crittenden MR, et al. OX40 signaling in head and neck squamous cell carcinoma: overcoming immunosuppression in the tumor microenvironment. Oral Oncol 2016;52:1–10.

65. Curti BD, Kovacsovics-Bankowski M, Morris N, et al. OX40 is a potent immune-stimulating target in late-stage cancer patients. Cancer Res 2013;73(24): 7189–98.

66. Jensen SM, Maston LD, Gough MJ, et al. Signaling through OX40 enhances antitumor immunity. Semin Oncol 2010;37(5):524–32.

67. Glisson BS, Leidner R, Ferris RL, et al. Phase 1 study of MEDI0562, a humanized OX40 agonist monoclonal antibody (mAb), in adult patients (pts) with advanced solid tumors. Ann Oncol 2016;27: vi361.

68. Cheuk AT, Mufti GJ, Guinn BA. Role of 4-1BB:4-1BB ligand in cancer immunotherapy. Cancer Gene Ther 2004;11(3):215–26.

69. Vinay DS, Kwon BS. Immunotherapy of cancer with 4-1BB. Mol Cancer Ther 2012;11(5):1062–70.

70. Mittler RS, Bailey TS, Klussman K, et al. Anti-4-1BB monoclonal antibodies abrogate T cell-dependent humoral immune responses in vivo through the induction of helper T cell anergy. J Exp Med 1999; 190(10):1535–40.

71. Segal NH, He AR, Doi T, et al. Phase I study of single-agent utomilumab (PF-05082566), a 4-1BB/CD137 agonist, in patients with advanced cancer. Clin Cancer Res 2018;24(8):1816–23.

72. Shenoy BV, Fort L 3rd, Benjamin SP. Malignant melanoma primary in lymph node. The case of the missing link. Am J Surg Pathol 1987;11(2):140–6.

73. Manouras A, Genetzakis M, Lagoudianakis E, et al. Malignant gastrointestinal melanomas of unknown origin: should it be considered primary? World J Gastroenterol 2007;13(29):4027–9.

74. Herbst RS, Soria JC, Kowanetz M, et al. Predictive correlates of response to the anti-PD-L1 antibody MPDL3280A in cancer patients. Nature 2014; 515(7528):563–7.

75. Spranger S, Spaapen RM, Zha Y, et al. Up-regulation of PD-L1, IDO, and $T_{regs}$ in the melanoma tumor microenvironment is driven by CD8[+] T cells. Sci Transl Med 2013;5(200):200ra116.

# Reconstruction of Head and Neck Melanoma Defects

Al Haitham Al Shetawi, MD, DMD[a,b,]*, Will Wing, DO[c]

## KEYWORDS

- Head and neck melanoma • Facial reconstruction • Local flaps • Regional flaps

## KEY POINTS

- Head and neck skin defects are usually reconstructed with local and regional flaps.
- Most of the local flaps used in head and neck defect restoration are random pattern flaps.
- The choice of flap relies on the wound characteristics such as size and depth, the anatomic features such as facial unit boundaries and skin quality, and the surgeon's creativity.

## INTRODUCTION

Skin cancer is the most common type of cancer in humans.[1] Melanoma only accounts for less than 2% of skin cancer cases but is the number one cause of skin cancer related deaths.[1] About 10% to 25% of melanoma is found in the head and neck region, commonly found in the face (40%–60%), neck (20%–29%), scalp (14%–49%), and the ear (8%–11%).[2] The mainstay of treatment of melanoma is complete surgical extirpation. Proper planning for defect reconstruction in the head and neck region is equally important to achieve the best possible aesthetic and functional outcome. There are many methods and techniques to repair defects in the head and neck region, including primary wound closure, skin grafts, and local and regional flaps. When considering the reconstructive technique, it is imperative to have good understanding of the tumor type and stage, nodal status, and the possible need for additional treatments in the future. In this paper the authors discuss the common flaps used in head and neck reconstruction for melanoma.

Flaps used for reconstruction are generally classified based on the arrangement of their blood supply, configuration, proximity to the defect, and method of transfer.[3] Local flaps are those located adjacent to or near the defect, regional flaps are located at a significant distance from the defect with preservation of the feeding vessels, and free flaps require division of the vessels and anastomosis.[3] Methods of transferring flaps can be broadly categorized into pivotal, advancement, and hinged flaps.[3] Most local flaps use a combination of pivoting and advancement, but the major mechanism used will determine the term given when describing a specific flap.

## PIVOTAL FLAPS

Pivotal flaps are local cutaneous flaps that can be further categorized into 3 different categories: rotational, transpositional, and interpolated. These flaps are rotated around a fixed pivotal point toward the defect. The fixed pivotal point creates an inverse relationship between the

a Division of Surgical Oncology, Department of Surgery, Vassar Brothers Medical Center, Nuvance Health, Dyson Center for Cancer Care, Poughkeepsie, NY 12601, USA; b Division of Oral & Maxillofacial Surgery, Department of Surgery, Vassar Brothers Medical Center, Nuvance Health, Poughkeepsie, NY 12601, USA; c Department of Surgery, Vassar Brothers Medical Center, Nuvance Health, 45 Reade Place, GME, 4th Floor, Poughkeepsie, NY 12601, USA
* Corresponding author. Surgical Oncology, Dyson Center for Cancer Care, Poughkeepsie, 45 Reade Place, 3rd Floor, NY 12601.
E-mail address: Al-haitham.al-shetawi@nuvancehealth.org

Oral Maxillofacial Surg Clin N Am 34 (2022) 283–298
https://doi.org/10.1016/j.coms.2021.11.002

degree in which the flap is rotated and the effective length of the flap.[4] There can be up to 40% loss in length when the flap is pivoted through an arc of 180°.[4] The greater degree in which the flap is rotated also increases the chance of a dog ear deformity.[4]

## Rotational Flaps

Rotational flaps are designed with a curvilinear configuration with its base adjacent to the defect. They usually have a random pattern blood supply but may be axial depending on the base of the flap.[4] They are useful in many regions in the head and neck including cheek, upper neck, glabella, and scalp. Incorporation of Burow's triangle at the distal end of the flap avoids formation of a dog ear deformity. When feasible the use of an inferiorly based flap can help promote lymphatic drainage and reduce flap edema.[4]

## Transpositional Flaps

Transpositional flaps are designed as rotational flaps but with a linear configuration, usually using a geometric shape. Typically, the border of the flap is also a border of the defect, but it can also be designed in such a way that only the base of the flap is contiguous with the defect.[4] It is a common flap used to reconstruct small to medium size head and neck skin defects. Transpositional flaps usually have a random pattern blood supply but occasionally will have an axial or a compound blood supply.[4] One of the most notable advantages to a transpositional flap is the variable distance at which the flap can be designed away from the defect.[4] By selecting areas of greater skin elasticity or redundancy, this can allow for better camouflage and aesthetic outcome of the donor site scar.

## Interpolated Flaps

Interpolated flaps are also designed with a linear configuration, but the base of the flap is not contiguous with the defect.[4] Transfer of the flap must cross an intact portion of the skin to reach the defect, which can be done in different techniques.[3] The first technique uses a pedicle that is deepithelialized and travels under a bridge of skin as an island flap; this allows a single-stage reconstruction.[3] The second technique uses a staged reconstruction. The flap is transferred over a skin bridge. After flap healing and formation of collateral blood supply from the recipient bed, a second stage is performed to section the connecting portion of the flap between the recipient bed and donor site.[3]

## ADVANCEMENT FLAPS

Advancement flaps are designed with a linear configuration and are transferred into the site of the defect by stretching it in a single vector.[4] For proper wound closure these flaps depend on the primary and secondary movement of the skin. Primary movement corresponds to the elasticity of the tissue of the flap itself, whereas secondary movement corresponds to the elasticity of the tissue adjacent to the defect. Advancement flaps can be further categorized into single or unipedicle, bipedicle, and V-Y.[3]

### Unipedicle and Bipedicle Flaps

Unipedicle advancement flaps use parallel incisions to allow one directional movement of the flap using a single vector toward the defect.[5] The flap is designed adjacent to the defect where one border of the defect is contiguous with a border of the flap.[4] Primary tissue movement is achieved by pushing or pulling the flap forward, whereas the tissue adjacent to the defect and flap move in the opposite direction, providing secondary movement. To create tension-free closure and avoid displacement of nearby facial structures, there must be adequate undermining of the advancement flap as well as the surrounding skin and soft tissue.[5]

Similar to pivotal flaps, a dog ear deformity may develop at the base of the flap. However, with unipedicle advancement flaps this tends to occur on both sides of the base of the flap. These deformities can be repaired using different techniques. They can be excised at the base or anywhere along the length of the flap using Burow's triangles or can be eliminated without excision with the use of bilateral Z-plasty at the base of the flap.[4] If there is sufficient length to the flap, the standing cutaneous deformities can also be corrected without excision and instead be corrected using proper suturing technique with closure; this is achieved by distributing it along the length of the flap creating smaller puckers of tissue and by sequentially suturing the wound lengths in one-half.[4]

Unipedicle advancement flaps are useful for facial defects on the forehead, particularly around the eyebrow and helical rim, the upper and lower lips, and the medial cheek. For large defects, bilateral unipedicle advancement flaps can be used for reconstruction. Depending on the configuration of the defect, an "H-" or a "T-"shaped repair or better known as H-plasty and T-plasty can be performed.[5] The flaps are designed on opposite sides of the defect and are advanced toward each other where each flap is repairing a portion of the defect.[4]

## V-Y Flaps

V-Y advancement flaps use a V-shaped flap that is advanced into the primary defect, leaving behind a secondary triangular donor defect. The secondary defect is repaired by advancing the 2 edges of the donor site wound together for primary closure of the donor defect.[4] This effectively makes a "Y" configuration on closure, hence the V-Y advancement flap. It is commonly used for defects in the cheek and upper lip region.[6]

## HINGE FLAPS

The hinge flap, sometimes referred to as trapdoor, turn-in, or turn-down flap, uses a linear or curvilinear design.[4] The base of the flap is on one border of the defect and is essentially turned over as the page of a book. It is useful in the reconstruction of facial defects that require internal and external lining surfaces, such as full-thickness nasal defects. The flap is raised in the subcutaneous tissue plane and turned over onto the defect where the epithelial surface of the flap provides the internal lining of the defect. A second flap is used to cover the subcutaneous surface of the hinge flap, providing external defect coverage. These flaps often have limited or restricted vascularity because they rely on the blood supply of the subcutaneous pedicle until they develop collateral blood supply from the recipient bed.[4] To enhance the vascularity of the flap and improve survival, it is recommended that when elevating the flap, the plane of dissection becomes deeper as the dissection proceeds toward the base of the flap.[4]

## DEFECTS OF THE SCALP

Repairing scalp defects can be challenging and the choice of reconstructive technique is affected by numerous factors including size and location of the defect, the quality of surrounding tissue, the presence or absence of periosteum, the presence or absence of hair, and patient comorbidities.[7] The location of the hairline is important to consider when planning a reconstruction. There

are a variety of local flaps that can be used to achieve an aesthetically pleasing outcome.

The 5 layers of the scalp can be remembered using the mnemonic SCALP: S, skin; C, subcutaneous tissue; A, aponeurosis (galea aponeurotica); L, loose areolar tissue; and P, pericranium. The galea aponeurotic is a dense fibrous sheet of connective tissue that serves as the strength layer of the scalp. It is contiguous with the anterior frontalis muscles, the posterior occipitalis muscles, and the bilateral temporoparietal fascia. The loose areolar tissue gives the scalp the ability to move. The inherent mobility of the scalp can be divided into tight and loose regions in relation to the underlying tissue.[8] Tight regions occur centrally where there is no muscle or fascia, whereas loose regions are more peripheral where these components are present.[8]

The scalp receives its blood supply from the internal and external carotid systems. The anterior scalp is supplied by the supraorbital and supratrochlear vessels. The lateral scalp is supplied by the superficial temporal vessels. The posterior scalp is supplied by the occipital vessels as well as perforators from the trapezius and splenius capitis.[8]

Techniques for scalp reconstruction can be broadly categorized into primary closure, healing by secondary intention, skin grafting, local and regional flaps, and free flaps. In this section the authors highlight the commonly used techniques to reconstruct defects after melanoma resection. Scalp defects that are amenable to primary closure require adequate tissue laxity for tension-free repair and tend to be small defects (Fig. 1). For scalp defects that are not amenable to primary repair, split skin grafts can be used (Fig. 2). Skin graft is a good option in bald patients. When using a skin graft to reconstruct a scalp defect, the pericranium should be preserved. Although not always feasible due to the required excision margins, preservation of pericranium can improve the take of a skin graft.[8] Skin grafts should be avoided in patients with history of radiation therapy to the scalp. When the skull is barren, skin grafts are not usually recommended for reconstruction, but

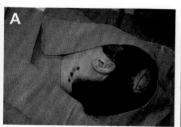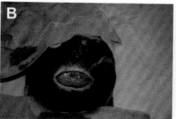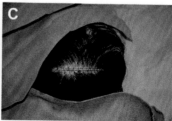

**Fig. 1.** Marking for excision (*A*), defect (*B*), and repair with primary closure (*C*).

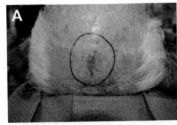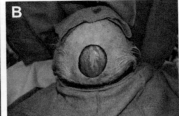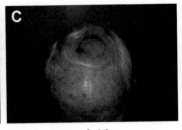

**Fig. 2.** Marking for excision (*A*), defect (*B*), and final outcome after split-thickness skin graft (*C*).

if deemed necessary, small drill holes can be done to create bleeding points to improve the likelihood of graft take.[8] Local flaps such as a transpositional, rotational, and O-Z flaps can be used for small to large scalp defects.

### Transpositional Flap

A transpositional flap has a linear configuration. It is usually a random pattern flap but may have an axial or a compound blood supply.[4] It is a common flap used for small to medium size scalp defects. One of the most notable advantages to a transpositional flap is the variable distance at which the flap can be designed away from the defect.[4] By selecting areas of greater skin elasticity or redundancy, this can allow for better camouflage and aesthetic outcome of the donor site scar (**Fig. 3**).

### Rotational Flap

A rotational flap has a curvilinear configuration with its base is adjacent to the defect.[4] It is usually a random pattern blood supply but may be an axial or a compound blood supply depending on the base of the flap.[4] It is a common flap used for medium to large scalp defects (**Fig. 4**).

### O-Z Flap

The O-Z flap is a double rotational flap that uses 2 opposing semicircular flaps around the diameter of a circular defect. Each flap is advanced, rotated, and fixed 90° from its incision point.[9] The flaps depend on the available surrounding tissue and

can be designed with equal or unequal lengths. The final closure creates a "Z" scar. Similar to the rotational flap, it has a random pattern blood supply. It is useful in medium to large scalp defects (**Fig. 5**).

## DEFECTS OF THE FOREHEAD

When feasible, primary repair of forehead defects provides good aesthetic outcome. The closure should be along the relaxed skin tension lines (**Fig. 6**). When the defect is not amenable to primary repair, local flaps provide good option. Consideration to the proximity of the hairline and eyebrows should be given when designing the flap to avoid distortion and poor aesthetic outcome.

### Bilateral Advancement Flap

The bilateral horizontal advancement flap or sometimes referred to as an "H-plasty" is useful for small to medium size defects in the central and lateral forehead.[10] It is designed with 2 opposing rectangular advancement flaps. The transverse incisions are made along the naturally occurring relaxed skin tension lines of the forehead, camouflaging the scars, and the vertical scar is only as big as the defect (**Fig. 7**). When elevating the flaps, care should be taken to avoid damage to the supratrochlear and or supraorbital nerve branches. Rose and colleagues recommend using up to a 2:1 length to width ratio when creating the flaps.[10]

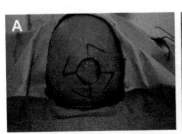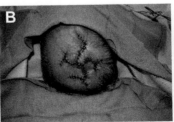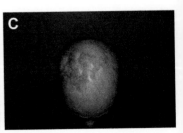

**Fig. 3.** Marking for the flap after excision (*A*), flap closure (*B*), and final outcome (*C*).

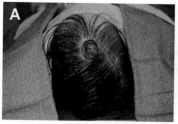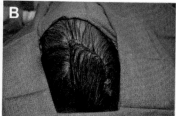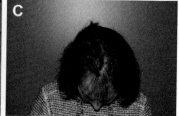

**Fig. 4.** Marking for the flap after excision (*A*), flap closure (*B*), and final outcome (*C*).

## Rhomboid Flap

The rhomboid flap is a random pattern transposition flap, also commonly called the "Limberg flap" after Alexander Limberg who first described the flap in 1945.[11] The mathematical principles of the rhomboid flap have been modified several times over, most notably by Lister and Gibson in the 1970s where they described using the classic angles of 60° and 120° with equal lengths on all sides.[12] The rhomboid flap was further modified by Quaba in 1987 in which he described using the basis of the Limberg flap to repair circular defects.[13]

The rhomboid flap is commonly used for small to medium size forehead defects but can also be used to cover relatively larger areas by using multiple rhomboids. The flap is moved laterally about a pivot point into the adjacent defect, and the donor defect is primarily closed (**Fig. 8**).

## Rotational Advancement Flap

The rotational flap is a good option for medium to large forehead defects. Ransom and Jacono described a double-opposing rotation advancement flap for closure of circular forehead defects in an attempt to avoid unappealing changes to the hairline or brow.[14] The flap has a random pattern blood supply and is pedicled on a wide base. For defects in the central forehead and anterior hairline the flaps may be raised in the subgaleal plane, and for defects in the lateral forehead the flaps are raised in the subcutaneous plane to protect the frontal branch of the facial nerve. This technique helps maintain the vertical height of the forehead[14] (**Fig. 9**).

## DEFECTS OF THE CHEEK

Cheek defects can be reconstructed with a variety of flaps. In general, cheek defects are preferably reconstructed with tissue from adjacent units such as the neck, submental area, or chest, using local or regional flaps to maintain skin color and texture.[15]

## Cervicofacial Flap

The cervicofacial flap was first described by Beare in 1969 for the reconstruction of orbital exenteration defects.[16] It has since been modified in

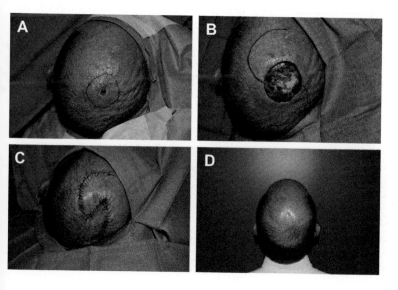

**Fig. 5.** Marking for excision (*A*), marking for the flap after excision (*B*), flap closure (*C*), and final outcome (*D*).

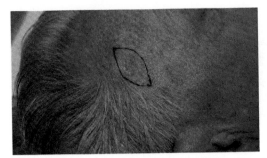

**Fig. 6.** Marking for primary repair along the relaxed skin tension lines.

various ways, most notably by Mustarde who described using the flap to reconstruct large defects of the periorbital region.[17] The flap can have a random pattern blood supply when raised in the subcutaneous layer or an axial blood supply when raised below the superficial musculoaponeurotic layers.[18] The latter would then be termed a myofasciocutaneous flap, and the blood supply would depend on the anterior or posterior position of the flap base. For an anterior based flap, the submental and perforating branches of the facial artery supply blood, and for a posterior based flap, the blood supply is from the perforators of the superficial temporal artery.[4] Raising the flap below the superficial musculoaponeurotic layer is typically used for larger defects, giving the flap a more robust blood supply and minimizing the risk of ischemia or venous congestion at the superior tip.[18] The cervicofacial flap can provide good skin color, thickness, and texture match for reconstruction of cheek defects, and the scars are well camouflaged (**Figs. 10** and **11**).

### The Submental Island Flap

The submental island flap was first described in 1993 by Martin and colleagues, giving a better alternative to free flap reconstruction of orofacial defects.[19] Three years later, Sterne and colleagues described using the flap in oral squamous cell carcinoma.[20] It has since become a popular choice for reconstruction of oral cavity defects,

oropharynx, hypopharynx, maxilla, parotid bed, chin, face, upper and lower lip, and neck. It is an axial pattern flap usually raised in an elliptical shape. The long dominant pedicle is based on the submental artery and can provide cutaneous dimensions up to 7 to 8 cm in width and 15 to 18 cm in length.[21] It has a wide arc of rotation extending from the medial canthus to the zygomatic arch. One of the potential disadvantages to this flap is the risk of venous congestion.[21] Overall, the submental island flap provides excellent matching of skin color, shape, and tissue texture to the original defect site, and the closure of the donor site leaves behind a well-hidden scar (**Fig. 12**).

### Nasolabial Flap

The first descriptions of the nasolabial flap can be traced back as far as 700 BC by Indian surgeon Sushruta who described it in his book entitled *Sushruta Samhita*.[22] It was traditionally used for alar reconstruction and has since been modified and described by many other surgeons for reconstruction of the nasal tip, dorsal, and columella, as well as intraoral reconstruction and cheek reconstruction.[23] Most nasolabial flaps have a random pattern blood supply but can also be raised as an axial flap based on the design with a superiorly or inferiorly based pedicle. Superiorly based flaps are supplied by the angular artery and are commonly used in the reconstruction of nasal defects or intraoral defects of the upper sulcus or palate.[4] Inferiorly based flaps are supplied by the facial artery and are commonly used for lower lip defects and defects in the floor of the mouth.[4] The design will depend on location of the defect and arc of rotation needed to reconstruct a defect in a tension-free manner. For facial defects the nasolabial flap can be used in the form of an advancement, rotational, or transposition flap.[24] The proximity to these defects, the similar color and texture of the skin from this flap, and using the nasolabial crease to hide the scar make it an advantageous flap for an aesthetically pleasing reconstruction (**Fig. 13**).

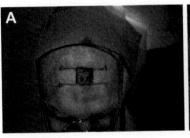
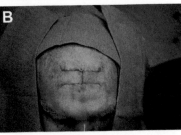

**Fig. 7.** Marking for the flap after excision (*A*) and flap closure (*B*).

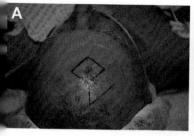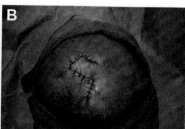

**Fig. 8.** Marking for excision and flap (*A*) and flap closure (*B*).

## DEFECTS OF THE NOSE

Defects of the nose can cause significant aesthetic deformity due to its central location in the face and 3-dimensional shape. Therefore, reconstruction of the nose is particularly challenging. As other facial defects, reconstruction of nasal defects can be achieved with primary closure, healing by secondary intention, skin grafting, and a variety of local and regional flaps. Some of the commonly used flaps are the bilobed flap, paramedian forehead flap, glabellar flap, and the nasolabial flap.

### Bilobed Flap

The bilobed flap is a random pattern double or sometimes triple transposition flap that was first described by Esser in 1918 for the repair of nasal defects.[25] Originally the flap was described to have a rotational arc of 180°. Esser described using 2 flaps of equal size at 90° and 180° from the axis of the defect. Zitelli later modified the flap design by limiting the total rotational arc to between 90° and 110°.[26] In Zitelli's description, the first flap is 45° from the axis of the defect and the second elongated flap is 90° to 110° from the

axis of the defect.[27] The Zitelli modification minimizes dog ear formation and reduces the risk of pincushion formation, significantly improving the cosmesis of the flap.[27] The first lobe of the flap is used to fill the primary defect and is usually the same size as the defect. The second lobe is adjacent to the first and is used to fill the secondary defect. The remaining defect from the secondary lobe is then closed primarily. The use of tissue adjacent to the defect allows the use of skin that is similar in color and texture and thus have a good cosmetic outcome (**Fig. 14**).

### Paramedian Forehead Flap

The use of the paramedian forehead flap for reconstruction of nasal amputation defects dates back as far as 1500 BC.[28] It later started to gain popularity in the United States with descriptions from Blair in 1925[29] and Kazanjian in 1946.[30] It was then further modified by Millard who described narrowing the base of the flap with a dependent blood supply from the supratrochlear vessels.[31] With his modification, the flap could be increased in length, and the narrower base allowed it to be

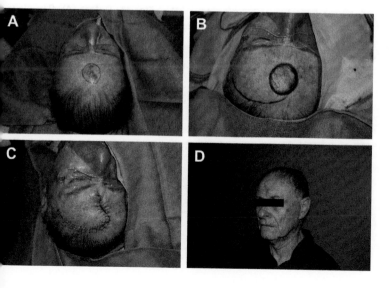

**Fig. 9.** Marking for excision (*A*), flap after excision (*B*), flap closure (*C*), and final outcome (*D*).

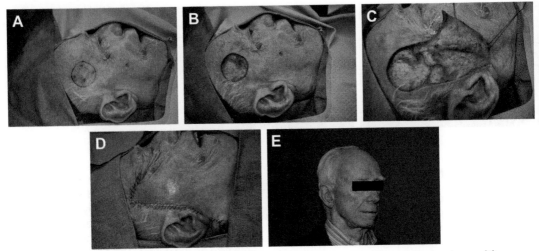

**Fig. 10.** Marking for excision (*A*), defect (*B*), flap elevation (*C*), flap closure (*D*), and final outcome (*E*).

more easily rotated onto the defect. It is an interpolated flap with an axial blood supply based on the supratrochlear artery and vein.[28] It is typically used in reconstruction of medium to large nose defects.[4] The texture, thickness, and similar skin color to surrounding tissue make the flap a very good option in reconstruction of these defects. The downside to its use is the need for a staged reconstruction (**Fig. 15**).

### Glabellar Flap

Reconstruction of defects using tissue from the glabellar region was first described by Carl von Graefe in 1818.[32] Since this first description, the glabellar flap has been modified by many other surgeons, making it a versatile flap to reconstruct

defects in the nasal region. It was originally described as a V-Y advancement flap used for defects in the upper third of the nose with a random pattern blood supply. Depending on the size and location of the defect it can also be raised as a transposition flap or V-Y rotation advancement flap as described by others.[32] The glabellar area is a source of redundant thick skin that can easily match the texture, consistency, and color of the defect. An advantage of the flap is that it can be done under local anesthesia, decreasing risk for patients who otherwise could not tolerate general anesthesia. Given the thick skin of the glabella as compared with the nose, this at times can affect the cosmetic outcome of the flap. To avoid mismatch of thickness of the flap and the

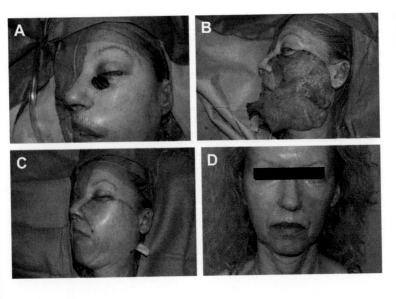

**Fig. 11.** Defect (*A*), flap elevation (*B*), flap closure (*C*), and final outcome (*D*).

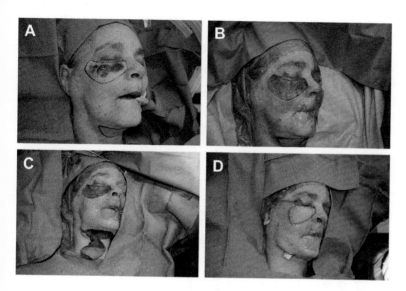

**Fig. 12.** Marking for excision (*A*), defect (*B*), flap elevation (*C*), and flap closure (*D*).

surrounding tissue, at the time of harvest the flap can be thinned by resecting most of the subcutaneous fatty tissue without fear of ischemia; this is because the flap has a stable network of vascular blood supply from perforators of the lateral nasal branch of the facial artery, the angular artery, and the dorsal nasal artery.[4] The secondary defect of this advancement flap is usually closed primarily, resulting in well-hidden scars (**Fig. 16**).

### Nasolabial Flap

Superiorly based flaps are supplied by the angular artery and are commonly used in the reconstruction of nasal defects.[24] The design will depend on location of the defect and arc of rotation needed. The proximity to the defect, the similar color and texture of the skin, and using the nasolabial crease to hide the scar make it an advantageous flap for an aesthetically pleasing reconstruction (**Fig. 17**).

### DEFECTS OF THE AURICLE

As the nose, the auricle plays an important role in appearance. Because of its complex 3-

dimensional shape, even small defects can be disfiguring. Reconstruction of small defects can be done with simple techniques such as wedge resection and skin grafting. However, for moderate to large size defects, a flap or a multistage operation might be necessary.

### Wedge Resection

The wedge resection is a useful approach to reconstructing small defects of the helix. For defects up to 1 cm, the wedge-shaped defect can be primarily closed with an adequately pleasing aesthetic result. In defects greater than 1 cm and up to 2 cm, closing the defect primarily without further modification may result in irregularities in form and contour of the auricle.[33] In 1886, Trendelenburg recommended the removal of Burow's triangles to avoid such results.[33] His technique has since been modified in many ways regarding the configuration and placement of the Burow's triangles. They are most often placed in the scapha or along the border between the concha and its transition to the antihelix. The auricle may be shortened slightly when using a wedge resection, but

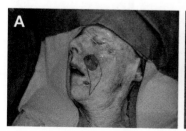
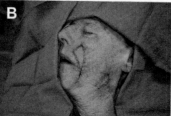
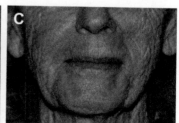

**Fig. 13.** Marking for the flap after excision (*A*), flap closure (*B*), and final outcome (*C*).

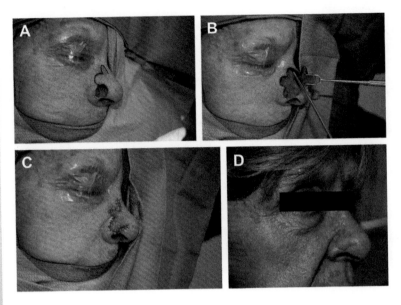

**Fig. 14.** Marking for flap after excision (*A*), flap elevation (*B*), flap closure (*C*), and final outcome (*D*).

it normally maintains the original contour[33] (**Fig. 18**).

## Rhomboid Flap

The rhomboid flap raised from the preauricular skin can be used to reconstruct small defects of the conchae. The preauricular flap incisions can be placed along the relaxed skin tension lines, resulting in well-camouflaged scars (**Fig. 19**). For earlobe defects, reconstruction can be done with 2 opposing flaps or a single bilobed double-over flap, still following the Limberg principles in flap configuration.[34]

## Trap Door Flap

The trap door flap was first described by Masson in 1972 for reconstruction of concha-helix defects.[35] It is a random pattern flap that is commonly used for conchal fossa defects. The flap is raised from the postauricular region with a pivotal axis in the postauricular groove, rotated forward 180° and inset to fill the conchal defect.[36]

The secondary defect is primarily closed and well hidden behind the auricle. Cosmetic outcomes are generally good, given the skin of the flap is similar in color and texture of the auricle (**Fig. 20**).

## Postauricular Flap

Postauricular flaps are useful in reconstruction of defects found in the upper, middle, and inferior postauricular and mastoid region.[37] They are commonly used for helical rim defects and generally give good cosmetic results, given the flap is similar in color, texture, and thickness to the skin of the auricle. It is a local advancement flap with a random pattern blood supply. Reconstruction is done in a 2-staged procedure.[33] The first stage is to create the flap and the second is to divide the flap (**Fig. 21**).

## Modified Gavello Flap

The bilobed flap is a random pattern double transposition flap that was first described by Esser in 1918 for the repair of nasal defects.[25] Gavello later

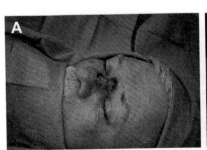
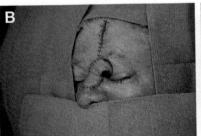
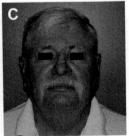

**Fig. 15.** Defect (*A*), flap closure (*B*), and final outcome (*C*).

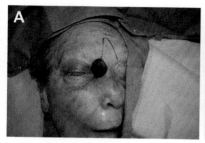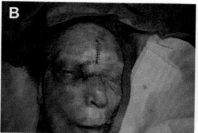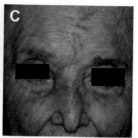

**Fig. 16.** Marking for flap after excision (*A*), flap closure (*B*), and final outcome (*C*).

modified this technique in the 1970s for reconstruction of the earlobe. It uses a horizontal bilobed flap that is inferior and posterior to the defect in the postauricular mastoid region.[38] The posterior flap is folded over behind the anterior flap. The secondary defect is closed by mobilizing the surrounding skin, or for larger defects, a cutaneous or cartilaginous graft can be used.[38] The flap is relatively simple and is a single stage procedure. It provides good cosmetic results with preservation of shape and volume of the earlobe (**Fig. 22**).

## DEFECTS OF THE NECK

Most small to medium size neck defects can be repaired by primary closure. Primary repair is feasible due to skin laxity and easy mobility. Primary repair in the neck usually heals with good cosmetic outcome if the repair is performed along the natural neck creases. Occasionally flaps need be used for larger defects.

### Keystone Flap

The keystone flap is a random pattern flap that was first described in 2003 by Dr Felix Behan.[39] He described the design as a curvilinear shaped trapezoid, which is essentially 2 conjoined V-Y advancement flaps in an end to side arrangement.[4] He further described 4 variations of the

flap depending on defect size, deep fascia division, use of a split-thickness skin graft to repair the secondary defect, degree of undermining, and use of double flap harvest.[40] Type I is typically used for smaller defects and uses direct closure.[40] Type II is when reconstruction takes place over a muscular compartment and the deep fascia on the outer compartment is divided to facilitate mobility of the flap[40]; this can be used with or without skin grafts. Type III is used for larger defects and uses a double island flap technique.[40] Type IV involves rotation and advancement of the flap. Up to 50% of the flap is elevated and rotated to close the defect with or without skin grafting.[40] This flap uses skin that is adjacent to the defect, providing excellent skin color and texture match to the surrounding skin (**Fig. 23**).

### Supraclavicular Artery Island Flap

Pallua and colleagues first described the supraclavicular artery island flap in 1997 for releasing post-burn mentosternal contractors.[41] With modification this flap has become popular in the reconstruction of the lower face and neck. It can also be used for pharyngeal reconstruction and for stomal defects.[42] The supraclavicular flap is a relatively easy flap to harvest and can even be used for reconstruction in patients who have had previous neck dissections. It is a local rotational

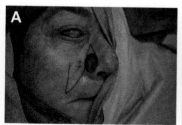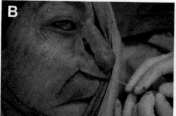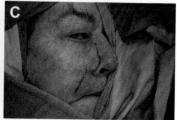

**Fig. 17.** Marking for the flap after excision (*A*), flap advancement (*B*), and closure (*C*).

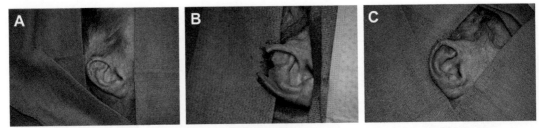

**Fig. 18.** Marking for excision(A), defect (*B*), and closure (*C*).

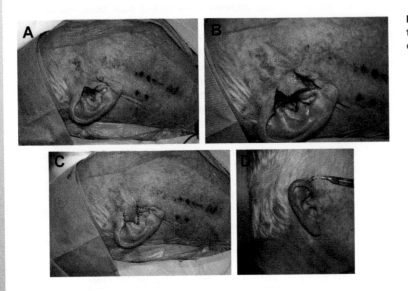

**Fig. 19.** Defect (*A*), flap elevation (*B*), closure (*C*), and final outcome (*D*).

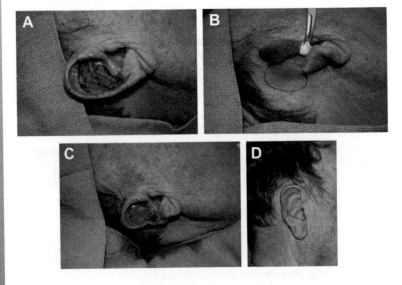

**Fig. 20.** Defect (*A*), flap marking (*B*), flap closure (*C*), and final outcome (*D*).

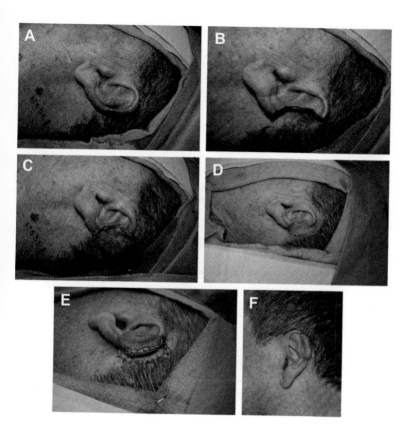

**Fig. 21.** Marking for excision (*A*), defect (*B*), flap closures (*C*), flap healing before division (*D*), flap division and skin graft (*E*), and final outcome (*F*).

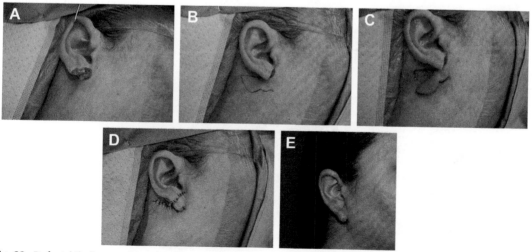

**Fig. 22.** Defect (*A*), flap marking (*B*), flap elevation (*C*), flap closure (*D*), and final outcome (*E*).

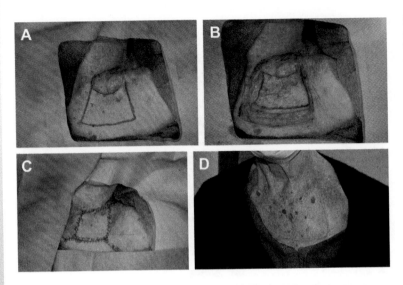

Fig. 23. Flap marking after excision (*A*), flap elevation (*B*), flap closure (*C*), and final outcome (*D*).

flap that is supplied by the supraclavicular artery, which is a branch from the transverse cervical artery.[42] It is recommended that the flap is not harvested beyond the insertion of the deltoid muscle where the tip of the flap will be more reliant on a random pattern of perfusion and thus susceptible to ischemia and subsequent necrosis[42]; this in turn restricts the length of the flap. Advantages of this flap is the similar skin color and texture match to the defect area, as well as the thinness of the flap when compared with regional musculocutaneous flaps (**Fig. 24**).

## SUMMARY/DISCUSSION

In this paper, the authors review the most common flaps used to reconstruct the different units in the head and neck region after melanoma extirpation. The rich blood supply in the head and neck region allows the reliable use of variety of flaps. The goal of a reconstructive technique is to restore cosmetics and preserve the function. Most of the flaps used in head and neck skin reconstruction are local and regional flaps and rely on random or axial blood supply.

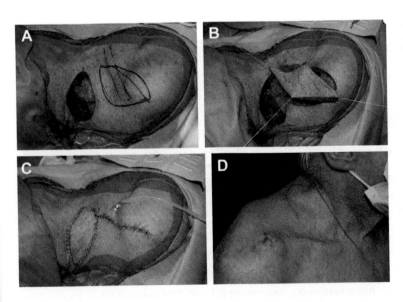

Fig. 24. Flap marking after excision (*A*), flap elevation (*B*), flap closure (*C*), and final outcome (*D*).

## CLINICS CARE POINTS

- Local flaps are preferred over other forms of flaps to restore head and neck skin defects. Local flaps provide excellent skin match with superior cosmetic outcome.

- When planning a flap for a melanoma defect, consideration should be made to the location of the incision for the sentinel lymph node. This is important in order to avoid compromising the blood supply to the planned flap.

- Every effort should be made to plan the resection margins and flap design along the facial unit boundaries to achieve the best possible aesthetic outcome.

## DISCLOSURE

No commercial of financial conflicts of interest for any authors.

## REFERENCES

1. Kimbrough Charles W, Urist Marshall M, McMasters Kelly M. Melanoma and Cutaneous Malignant Neoplasms. In: Townsend Courtney M, Beauchamp Daniel, Evers B Mark, Mattox Kenneth L, editors. Sabiston textbook of surgery: the biological basis of modern surgical practice. 20th edition. Philadelphia: Elsevier; 2017. p. 724–51.

2. Zito Patrick M, Scharf Richard. Melanoma of The Head And Neck. Treasure Island, FL: StatPearls Publishing; 2021. Available at: pubmed.ncbi.nlm.nih.gov/30020620/.

3.. Fernandes Rui. Flap Classification. In: Local and Regional Flaps in Head & Neck Reconstruction: A Practical Approach. Hoboken, NJ: John Wiley & Sons Inc; 2014. p. 2–4.

4. Baker Shan B. Reconstruction of Facial Defects. In: Flint Paul W, Fancis Howard W, Haughey Bruce H, Lesperance Marci M, Lund Valerie J, Robbins K Thomas, Thomas J Regan, editors. Cummings Otolaryngology: Head and Neck Surgery. 7th. Philadelphia: Elsevier; 2021. p. 311–30.

5. Shew Matthew, Kriet John David, Humphrey Clinton D. Flap basics II: Advancement Flaps. Facial Plastic Surgery Clinics 2017;25(3):323–35. https://doi.org/10.1016/j.fsc.2017.03.005.

6. Fernandes Rui. V to Y Advancement Flap. In: Local and Regional Flaps in Head & Neck Reconstruction: A Practical Approach. Hoboken, NJ: John Wiley & Sons Inc.; 2014. p. 50–6.

7. Leedy Jason E, Janis Jeffrey E, Rohrich Rod J, et al. Reconstruction of Acquired Scalp Defects: An Algorithmic Approach. Plastic and Reconstructive Surgery 2005;116(4):54–72. https://doi.org/10.1097/01.prs.0000179188.25019.6c.

8. Fernandes Rui. Scalp Reconstruction. In: Local and Regional Flaps in Head & Neck Reconstruction: A Practical Approach. Hoboken, NJ: John Wiley & Sons Inc.; 2014. p. 222–42.

9. Buckingham Edward D, Quinn Francis B, Calhoun Karen H. Optimal Design of O-to-Z Flaps for Closure of Facial Skin Defects. Archives of Facial Plastic Surgery 2003;5(1):92–5. https://doi.org/10.1001/archfaci.5.1.92.

10. Rose Victoria, Overstall Simon, Moloney Dphil Dominique, et al. The H-Flap: a useful flap for forehead reconstruction. British Journal of Plastic Surgery 2001;54(8):705–7. https://doi.org/10.1054/bjps.2001.3689.

11. Limberg AA. Mathematical Principles of Local Plastic Surgery Procedures on the Surface of the Human Body. Leningrad, Russia: Medgis; 1946.

12. Lister GD, Gibson T. Closure of rhomboid skin defects: the flaps of Limberg and Dufourmentel. British Journal of Plastic Surgery 1972;25(3):300–14. https://doi.org/10.1016/s0007-1226(72)80067-5.

13. Fernandes Rui. Rhomboid Flap. In: Local and Regional Flaps in Head & Neck Reconstruction: A Practical Approach. Hoboken, NJ: John Wiley & Sons Inc.; 2014. p. 12–9.

14. Ransom Evan R, Jacono Andrew A. Double-Opposing Rotation-Advancement Flaps for Closure of Forehead Defects. Archives of Facial Plastic Surgery 2012;14(5):342–5. https://doi.org/10.1001/archfacial.2012.7.

15. Al Shetawi Al Haitham, Quimby Anastasiya, Fernandes Rui. The Cervicofacial Flap in Cheek Reconstruction: A Guide for Flap Design. Journal of Oral Maxillofacial Surgery 2017;75(12):2708.e1–6. https://doi.org/10.1016/j.joms.2017.08.006.

16. Beare Robin. Flap Repair Following Exenteration of the Orbit. Proceedings of the Royal Society of Medicine 1969;62:1087–90.

17. Mustarde John C. The Use of Flaps in the Orbital Region. Plastic and Reconstructive Surgery 1970;45:146–50.

18. Fernandes Rui. Cervicofacial Advancement Flap. In: Local and Regional Flaps in Head & Neck Reconstruction: A Practical Approach. Hoboken, NJ: John Wiley & Sons Inc.; 2014. p. 92–102.

19. Martin D, Pascal JF, Baudet J, et al. The Submental Island Flap: A New Donor Site. Anatomy and Clinical Applications as a Free or Pedicled Flap. Plastic and Reconstructive Surgery 1993;92:867–73.

20. Sterne GD, Januszkiewicz JS, Hall PN, et al. The Submental Island Flap. British Journal of Plastic Surgery 1996;49(2):85–9. https://doi.org/10.1016/S0007-1226(96)90078-8.

21. Fernandes Rui. Submental Island Flap. In: Local and Regional Flaps in Head & Neck Reconstruction: A Practical Approach. Hoboken, NJ: John Wiley & Sons Inc.; 2014. p. 103–13.

22. Schmidt Brian L, Dierks Eric J. The Nasolabial Flap. Oral Maxillofacial Surgery Clinics of North America 2003;15(4):487–95. https://doi.org/10.1016/S1042-3699(03)00063-3.

23. Weathers William M, Wolfswinkel Erik M, Nguyen Huy, et al. Expanded Uses for the Nasolabial Flap. Seminars in Plastic Surgery 2013;27(2):104–9. https://doi.org/10.1055/s-0033-1351234.

24. Fernandes Rui. Nasolabial Flap. In: Local and Regional Flaps in Head & Neck Reconstruction: A Practical Approach. Hoboken, NJ: John Wiley & Sons Inc.; 2014. p. 41–9.

25. Esser JFS. Gestielte lokale Nasenplastik mit zweizipfligem Lappen, Deckung des sekundären Defektes vom ersten Zipfel durch den zweiten. Deutsche Zeitschrift für Chirugie 1918;143:385–90. https://doi.org/10.1007/BF02793149.

26. Zitelli John A. The Bilobed Flap for Nasal Reconstruction. Archives of Dermatology 1989;125(7):957–9. https://doi.org/10.1001/archderm.1989.01670190091012.

27. Fernandes Rui. Bilobed Flap. In: Local and Regional Flaps in Head & Neck Reconstruction: A Practical Approach. Hoboken, NJ: John Wiley & Sons Inc.; 2014. p. 5–11.

28. Fernandes Rui. Paramedian Forehead Flap. In: Local and Regional Flaps in Head & Neck Reconstruction: A Practical Approach. Hoboken, NJ: John Wiley & Sons Inc.; 2014. p. 62–74.

29. Blair Vilray P. Total and Subtotal Restoration of the Nose. JAMA 1925;85(25):1931–5. https://doi.org/10.1001/jama.1925.02670250005002.

30. Kazanjian VH. The Repair of Nasal Defects with Median Forehead Flap; Primary Closure of Forehead Wound. Plastic and Reconstructive Surgery 1947;2(2):184. https://doi.org/10.1097/00006534-194703000-00026.

31. Millard DR. Total Reconstructive Rhinoplasty and a Missing Link. Plastic and Reconstructive Surgery 1966;37(3):167–83. https://doi.org/10.1097/00006534-196602000-00022.

32. Koch Cody A, Archibald David J, Friedman Oren. Glabellar Flaps in Nasal Reconstruction. Facial Plastic Surgery Clinics of North America 2011;19(1):113–22. https://doi.org/10.1016/j.fsc.2010.10.003.

33. Weerda Hilko. Surgery of the Auricle: Tumors-Trauma-Defects-Abnormalities. New York, NY: Thieme; 2007.

34. Singh A, Singh G. Earlobe reconstruction using a Limberg flap in six ears. British Journal of Plastic Surgery 2003;56(1):33–6. https://doi.org/10.1016/S0007-1226(03)00002-X.

35. Masson JK. A simple island flap for reconstruction of concha-helix defects. British Journal of Plastic Surgery 1972;25(4):399–403. https://doi.org/10.1016/s0007-1226(72)80083-3.

36. Lynch J, Mahajan AL, Regan P. The trap door flap for reconstructing defects of the concha. British Journal of Plastic Surgery 2003;56(7):709–11. https://doi.org/10.1016/s0007-1226(03)00307-2.

37. Cerci Felipe B. Staged retroauricular flap for helical reconstruction after MOHS micrographic surgery. Anais Brasileiros De Dermatologia 2016;91(5 Suppl 1):144–7. https://doi.org/10.1590/abd1806-4841.20164733.

38. Cabral Ana Rita, Alonso Neide, Brinca Ana, et al. Earlobe reconstruction by the Gavello technique and bilobed flap. Anais Brasileiros De Dermatologia 2013;88(2):272–5. https://doi.org/10.1590/S0365-05962013000200018.

39. Behan Felix C. The Keystone Design Perforator Island Flap in reconstructive surgery. ANZ Journal of Surgery 2003;73(3):112–20. https://doi.org/10.1046/j.1445-2197.2003.02638.x.

40. Fernandes Rui. Keystone Flap. In: Local and Regional Flaps in Head & Neck Reconstruction: A Practical Approach. Hoboken, NJ: John Wiley & Sons Inc.; 2014. p. 57–61.

41. Pallua N, Machens HG, Rennekampff O, et al. The Fasciocutaneous Supraclavicular Artery Island Flap for Releasing Postburn Mentosternal Contractures. Plastic and Reconstructive Surgery 1997;99(7):1878–84. https://doi.org/10.1097/00006534-199706000-00011.

42. Fernandes Rui. The Supraclavicular Artery Island Flap. In: Local and Regional Flaps in Head & Neck Reconstruction: A Practical Approach. Hoboken, NJ: John Wiley & Sons Inc.; 2014. p. 147–61.

# Management of Head and Neck Mucosal Melanoma

Pablo Nenclares, MD[a,b,*], Kevin J. Harrington, PhD[a,b]

## KEYWORDS

- Head and neck mucosal melanoma • Molecular biology • Surgery • Radiotherapy • Immunotherapy
- Targeted therapy

## KEY POINTS

- The only potentially curative option is complete surgical resection with negative margins, but extensive surgery should be weighed against operative morbidity and high risk of recurrent disease.
- Postoperative radiotherapy may improve local/locoregional control, but there is no evidence that it improves overall survival.
- Adjuvant systemic therapy following radical primary surgery should be considered, including immunotherapy and targeted treatments where an appropriate mutation is present.
- Palliative systemic therapy for unresectable and metastatic HNMM includes immunotherapy with immune checkpoint inhibitors and targeted treatments (BRAF/MEK inhibitors and KIT inhibitors).
- Clinical trials for patients with HNMM remain a key priority.

## INTRODUCTION

First described by Weber in 1859, head and neck mucosal melanomas (HNMMs) are aggressive and rare malignancies from melanocytic origin. HNMMs account for 0.03% of all cancers and 1% to 4% of all melanomas but up to 60% of all mucosal melanoma. HNMMs involve the sinonasal cavities, oral cavity, pharynx, larynx, and upper esophagus.[1] HNMMs are usually associated with poor clinical outcomes despite aggressive treatment, mainly due to poor distant control.[2]

This article aims to present an update on pathobiological and management aspects of HNMM, focusing on the new perspectives given by the advent of systemic therapies such as targeted and immune therapies. Melanomas involving the eye are outside the scope of this review.

## CAUSE AND EPIDEMIOLOGY

HNMMs originate from melanocytes in the upper aerodigestive tract. Melanocytes are melanin-producing cells originating from the neural crest that migrate during development as neurocristic derivatives in endodermal or ectodermal mucosa.[3] The physiologic functions of melanocytes are not fully understood, but they seem to have a role in protection from reactive oxygen species, as stress sensors having the capacity to react to and to produce a variety of cytokines and growth factors, modulating immune, inflammatory, and antibacterial responses, and as neuroendocrine cells producing local neurotransmitters.[4]

Unlike cutaneous melanomas, HNMMs are not associated with sun exposure. To date, the cause of HNMMs is unknown and no risk factor has been clearly identified. The close proximity of commonly affected head and neck mucosal sites (lower nasal cavity, and maxillary sinuses, hard palate, and upper gingiva) has led some groups to suggest that the pathogenesis of these HNMMs is linked to abnormalities in embryonic development.[5] Exposure to inhaled and ingested carcinogens, particularly formaldehyde, has been suspected but not confirmed in several studies, and smoking may constitute a predisposing factor essentially for mucosal melanoma of the oral cavity.[6,7]

[a] Head and Neck Unit, The Royal Marsden Hospital, London, UK; [b] Division of Radiotherapy and Imaging, Targeted Therapy Team, The Institute of Cancer Research, 237 Fulham Road, London SW3 6JB, United Kingdom
* Corresponding author. Division of Radiotherapy and Imaging, Targeted Therapy Team, The Institute of Cancer Research, 237 Fulham Road, London SW3 6JB, United Kingdom
E-mail address: pablo.nenclares@icr.ac.uk

Oral Maxillofacial Surg Clin N Am 34 (2022) 299–314
https://doi.org/10.1016/j.coms.2021.11.008
1042-3699/22/

Patients' age at the time of diagnosis ranges between 30 and 90 years, with higher incidence in the sixth decade.[8] Most series describe a similar distribution between men and women, although some compilations have described a slight predominance in males.[9] There are some geographic differences concerning the incidence of mucosal melanoma in different countries and races. In Japan, oral mucosal melanomas account for 7.5% of all melanomas and 35% of all mucosal melanomas compared with less than 1% and 3.6%, respectively, for white Eropean background.[10] This higher percentage can possibly be attributed to the lower incidence of cutaneous melanoma in Japan. However, some investigators suspect a hereditary and environmental role in the pathogenesis.

## BIOLOGICAL CHARACTERISTICS AND MOLECULAR BIOLOGY

Several attempts have been made to understand the genetic alterations that underpin the development of HNMMs with the aim of identifying potential therapeutic targets. The malignant transformation of melanocytes occurs through sequential accumulation of genetic and molecular alterations. Several pathways are involved in primary clonal alteration, including the induction of cell proliferation, circumvention of cell senescence, and reduction of apoptosis.

There is substantial evidence that hyperactive receptor tyrosine kinase (RTK) signaling mediates the development and progression of melanoma.[11] c-KIT is one of the RTK that influences proliferation, migration, and survival of melanocytes. c-KIT is encoded by the proto-oncogene KIT and is activated by its ligand, stem cell factor (SCF), during melanogenesis. The binding of SCF to c-KIT leads to dimerization and autophosphorylation of tyrosine residues located in the intracellular part of the receptor (Fig. 1). It is well characterized that c-KIT phosphorylation triggers the activation of Src family kinases, which subsequently activates the mitogen-activated protein kinase (MAPK) pathway, involving the prosurvival and antiapoptotic Ras-Raf-Mek-Erk cascade.[12] In addition, the phosphatidylinositide-3-kinase (PI3K) survival pathway is switched on by phosphorylation of c-KIT.[13] Moreover, c-KIT tyrosine kinase receptor regulates the activity of MITF (microphthalmia-associated transcription factor).[14] MITF is a basic helix-loop-helix leucine zipper transcription factor that is essential for melanogenesis and melanocyte function due to its regulatory role in melanoblast and melanocyte proliferation, survival, differentiation, apoptosis,

and cell cycle arrest. Thus, c-KIT activation, independent of its ligand, through oncogenic mutations enables the receptor to phosphorylate various substrate proteins that leads to activation of signal transduction cascades that regulate cell proliferation, apoptosis, chemotaxis, and adhesion.[15]

In contrast with cutaneous melanoma wherein KIT mutations are rarely found, alterations in the KIT gene play an important oncogenic role in the development of mucosal melanomas. In 2006, Curtin and colleagues[16] noted KIT aberrations (21% KIT mutations, 61% c-KIT overexpression) in 15 (39%) of 38 cases of mucosal melanoma. This observation was confirmed in later publications, which reported alterations in the KIT gene in between 7% and 27% of HNMMs.[17–20] A recent publication of whole-exome sequencing analysis of 67 mucosal melanomas noted KIT mutations on 10 patients (15%).[21] Most KIT mutations in mucosal melanomas are detected in the juxtamembrane region of KIT encoded by exons 11 and 13, presumably resulting in the constitutive activation of c-KIT by promoting KIT dimerization in the absence of SCF or by preventing KIT from maintaining its autoinhibited conformation.

BRAF is a downstream effector within the MAPK signaling pathway, which in turn is one of the most important pathways in the regulation of cell growth, proliferation, differentiation, and apoptosis in all cells. BRAF mutations are highly prevalent (59%) in cutaneous melanomas.[22] Nearly 90% of reported BRAF alterations are oncogenic mutations that lie in the region that encodes the kinase domains, in which valine is replaced by glutamic acid at codon 600 (V600E).[23] However, BRAF mutations are significantly less frequent in melanomas on sun-protected skin such as acral melanomas and mucosal melanomas.[24] Pooling all the available literature, the rate of BRAF mutations in HNMMs lies between 3% and 15%. Moreover, BRAF mutations described in mucosal melanoma are diverse, but most of them are in the protein tyrosine kinase domain and most target the 594- to 600-amino acid hotspot region.[21] Approximately 10% to 20% of melanomas activate the MAPK pathway by mutation of NRAS, but mutations of both NRAS and BRAF virtually never occur together.[25] Reported NRAS mutation rate in HNMM ranges between 12% and 22% and usually involves codon 61, which is the dominant hotspot in cutaneous melanoma, and codons 12 and 13, both less commonly mutated in cutaneous melanoma.[26,27]

Alterations in the CDKN2A locus, encoding the tumor suppressor protein p16/INK4A, are frequently present in familial cases of cutaneous melanoma. CDKN2A/CDK4/6/CyclinD1 complex

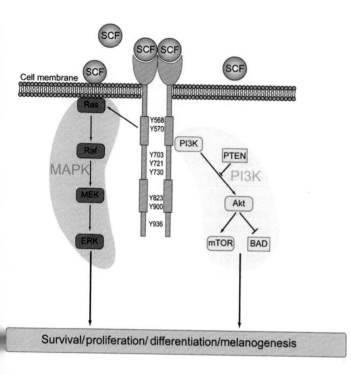

**Fig. 1.** c-KIT intracellular signaling pathway. (*From* Carlino MS, Todd JR, Rizos H. Resistance to c-Kit inhibitors in melanoma: insights for future therapies. Oncoscience. 2014 Jun 6;1(6):423–6.)

Survival/proliferation/differentiation/melanogenesis

is the essential regulator of cell cycle.[28] CDK4/6/CyclinD1 complex phosphorylates the retinoblastoma (Rb) and inhibits its activity, leading to the transition of G1 to S phase. By contrast, CDKN2A negatively regulates the progression of cell cycle via p16/INK4A phosphorylation of CDK4/6. Loss of p16 expression, CDKN2A mutations, and loss of heterozygosity are observed in up to 50% of mucosal melanomas, especially in oral mucosal melanomas in patients of East Asian ancestry.[21]

## PATHOLOGY AND PATHWAYS OF SPREAD

HNMMs are usually diagnosed at advanced stages, and they usually present macroscopically as aggressive nodular neoplasms with a vertical growth invading the underlying mucosa. The detection of *in situ* components is more challenging in the head and neck mucosa because of the thinness of the surface epithelium and their frequent ulceration.[29] Three patterns are recognized: *in situ*, in which the neoplasm remains restricted to the epithelial-connective tissue interface; deeply invasive or nodular pattern characterized by the breach of the basal membrane and invasion of the submucosa forming nodular aggregates; and a combination of both in which nodular component occurs together with an *in situ* or a radial growth pattern. This phase of radial growth is characterized by proliferation of atypical

melanocytes within the mucosa and by small breaches of the basement membrane with nests of invading cells and reactive inflammatory infiltrate in the most superficial part of the lamina propria. HNMMs may also present as multifocal lesions.[30,31]

HNMMs do not fit well into the classical classification for cutaneous melanoma due to the differing structures of the mucosal lamina propria and submucosa, compared with the dermis. Therefore, the histopathological classification and staging of cutaneous melanoma using Breslow thickness and Clark levels is not of use. On the contrary, Prasad and colleagues[32] proposed a classification system based on the level of invasion by the neoplasm comprising level 1 (*in situ*), level 2 (superficially invasive), and level 3 (deeply invasive). This classification functions as a predictor of survival, wherein level 3 tumors present the worst outcome.[32]

Histologically, mucosal melanomas are formed by medium- to large-sized cells that may be rounded, fusiform, polyhedral, epithelioid, spindle, desmoplastic, pleomorphic, microcytic, or a mixture of them, usually showing nuclei with one or multiple eosinophilic nucleoli. Tumors with mixed cell phenotypes have been found to be more aggressive and associated with a higher prevalence of vascular invasion and distant metastases.[33] Cancer cells may grow solid, loosely cohesive, storiform, pseudoalveolar, or forming organoid patterns. Mitotic activity is usually prominent. Most HNMMs contain some intracytoplasmic brown pigment, which should be confirmed as melanin. However, up to one-third can be amelanotic, which may represent a challenge for the pathologist as the variety of cell phenotypes can resemble other malignant neoplasms including poorly differentiated carcinoma, sarcoma, or lymphoma. Once the possibility of HNMM has been considered based on histopathological features, immunohistochemistry is a significant help in the diagnosis. HNMMs express S-100 protein and melanocytic markers including MART-1/Melan-A, tyrosinase, HMB-45, and MITF.[34] Malignant melanoma also reacts with antivimentin and NK1/C-3 antibodies, but not with antikeratin and antileukocytic antigen antibodies.[35]

Following confirmatory diagnosis, molecular analysis for mutations in BRAF and KIT should be performed routinely at the time of first diagnosis because the finding of any of these genomic alterations may offer patients therapeutic options. In the metastatic setting, it is recommended to perform molecular analyses from a metastatic sample (if available), because it represents the most recent lesion, and it is often composed by a large majority of neoplastic cells.

Hematological and lymphatic dissemination are common and early events. The profuse vascularization of the head and neck region, and especially the oral cavity, may influence the elevated incidence of metastasis. A retrospective multicenter study of 706 patients with mucosal melanomas found that up to 44% of all patients presented with metastatic disease at either regional sites (21.5%) or distant locations (23%).[36] The patterns of spread may vary for different primary sites. Patients with primary oral and laryngeal mucosal melanoma present higher incidence of regional nodal disease and lung metastases compared with patients with melanomas at other sites. Other common sites of metastatic spread include the liver, bone, and brain.[37,38]

## CLINICAL MANIFESTATIONS
### Head and Neck Mucosal Melanomas of the Nasal Cavity and Paranasal Sinuses

HNMMs occur most frequently in the nasal cavity, where the lateral nasal wall and nasal septum are the most common sites of origin. The maxillary antrum is the most commonly affected paranasal sinus, followed by the ethmoid, frontal, and sphenoid sinuses.[5,39] These tumors are associated with late presentation because they can be largely asymptomatic in early stages.[40]

The most common presenting complaints are nasal obstruction and epistaxis. Other symptoms include rhinorrhoea, pain or facial pressure, and lacrimation if there is invasion of the inferior meatus and the lacrimal duct. More advanced disease may present in the form of malar swelling, nasal deformity, proptosis, diplopia or neurologic symptoms.[41,42]

### Head and Neck Mucosal Melanomas of the Oral Cavity

Around 20% of HNMMs arise from the oral cavity, where the majority occur in the mucosa of the upper maxillary alveolar ridge and the hard palate. Most are initially asymptomatic, but those that present with symptoms usually cause pain, swelling, bleeding, and ill-fitting dentures. Visible oral lesions are macular or nodular, usually asymmetrical, with brown and black pigmentation, although up to 30% can be amelanotic. Nodular lesions are usually exophytic and ulcerated, and satellite lesions can be commonly seen on the hard palate and the maxillary or mandibular alveolus. Lesions arising from the alveolar ridge and hard palate favor early invasion of the underlying bone. Up to 25% of patients with oral mucosal melanomas may present with lymph node metastases.[43,44]

### Head and Neck Mucosal Melanomas of Other Sites

Primary pharyngeal, laryngeal, and upper esophageal mucosal melanomas are very uncommon. The most frequently affected region is the supraglottis, followed by the glottis. Their typical clinical presentation includes hoarseness, hemoptysis, dysphagia, and airway obstruction and, in these regards, they are indistinguishable from other laryngeal epithelial malignancies. In the pharynx, HNMMs may result in voice alterations, bleeding, and breathing and swallowing impairments. Symptoms of nasopharyngeal mucosal melanomas are similar to those of sinonasal melanomas, usually presenting with epistaxis, nasal obstruction, and obstruction of the Eustachian tube causing serous otitis. Together with oral mucosal melanomas, laryngeal melanomas present a high incidence of lymph node metastasis.[31,45]

## PATIENT EVALUATION AND STAGING

A comprehensive history with an emphasis on head and neck–related symptoms should be taken for all patients with suspected head and neck malignancies, and a detailed physical examination of the upper aerodigestive tract and neck should be performed. Neurologic examination including evaluation of eye movement and function and assessment of cranial nerves (particularly cranial nerves III, IV, V, and VI) is indicated.

The workup should include imaging evaluation and biopsy confirmation. Ideally, and when practical, imaging should precede biopsy because the image quality will not be confounded by post-biopsy artifacts and it enables a better evaluation of the tumor base and evaluation of the deep margins. Imaging assessment of the primary site should include contrast-enhanced cross-sectional imaging (either computed tomography [CT] or magnetic resonance imaging [MRI]) of the head and neck region. Dual modality assessment of the primary tumor with both CT and MRI should be considered, especially in cases with potential orbital and base of skull involvement or perineural spread. HNMMs tend to exhibit low-signal intensity on T2-weighted images and enhancement on precontrast T1-weighted images.[46,47]

Following imaging, a representative diagnostic biopsy should be performed. An adequate biopsy should incorporate adjacent clinically normal mucosa and extend into the submucosal tissues. For lesions with a high degree of suspicion of malignant melanoma, an incisional biopsy rather than an excisional biopsy is preferred to allow for subsequent appropriate surgical management. For patients who present with palpable cervical lymphadenopathy, pathologic confirmation by fine-needle aspiration or core biopsy of the suspicious lymph node is recommended.

Given the high rates of distant disease at presentation, systemic staging is considered mandatory at diagnosis[38] it should include contrast-enhanced CT scan of the thorax, abdomen, and pelvis and contrast-enhanced MRI or CT scan of the brain. The role of 18-fluorodeoxyglucose positron emission tomography (18-FDG PET) in the evaluation of mucosal melanomas is not completely established. Melanoma cells are known to be extremely FDG avid, and studies evaluating the overall accuracy of PET and PET/CT in primary mucosal melanomas at diagnosis or relapse have shown a high sensitivity and specificity in the detection of regional and distant metastasis, except for brain metastases.[48] Thus, PET/CT scan may be an alternative to whole-body contrast-enhanced CT scan in the regional and systemic staging.

Several staging systems have been proposed, most notably, those of Ballentyne and colleagues[49] and the modified version suggested by Prasad and colleagues.[32] Ballentyne and colleagues[49] described a simplified staging system that classifies HNMMs into the following 3 stages:

stage I for localized lesions, stage II for regional dissemination (cervical lymph node metastasis), and stage III for distant metastases. Although the advantage of this system lies in its simplicity, it offers extremely limited prognostic information for most patients. Prasad and colleagues[32] proposed the previously mentioned histology-derived staging system based on the invasion of tissue compartments within the mucosa. This system showed prognostic significance and difference in the survival rate for levels 1, 2, and 3 (5-year disease-specific survival rates of 75%, 52%, and 23%, respectively) but can only be determined after surgery.[32] In 2010, the American Joint Cancer Committee (AJCC) included specific chapters on HNMMs for the first time. Comparative studies have shown that AJCC/TNM have more precise value than previous systems.[50] The recently published eighth edition of the TNM has been adopted by the International Collaboration of Cancer Reporting (ICCR) and should be used as the main staging system for patients with HNMM because it shares the same terminology for the staging of other malignancies, and it reflects the prognosis of these patients. It is important to note that T1 or T2 categories do not exist and that all HNMMs are classified as either T3 or T4. In addition, the overwhelmingly poor prognosis of this malignancy is reflected by the fact that all HNMMs are classified as stage III or IV (**Table 1**).

## PRIMARY TREATMENT
### Surgery

Complete wide local excision with clear margins remains the mainstay of HNMM management. The therapeutic strategy should be tailored individually according to tumor extension, primary site, previous treatments, expected morbidities, and patient preferences. Whenever possible, wide and radical surgical procedures are attempted to obtain clear margins. There is mounting evidence that negative resection margins confer better local control and improved survival rates.[51] However, the ability to achieve a clear margin of excision should be weighed against the anticipated morbidity of more extensive surgery. Indeed, histopathologically assessed spread usually seems to be greater than the macroscopic extent of gross disease and, owing to the need to preserve vital structures, free surgical margins may not be achievable in some cases.[42]

A detailed description of the different potential surgical approaches is beyond the scope of this article, and the same principles and surgical techniques for excision of primary carcinomas of the head and neck region apply for HNMMs. For

**Table 1**
**American Joint Cancer Committee staging (eighth edition) for mucosal melanomas**

| AJCC/TNM 8th Edition for HNMMs | |
|---|---|
| **T: Primary tumor** | |
| pTx | Primary tumor cannot be, or has not been, assessed |
| T3 | Tumors limited to the mucosa and immediately underlying soft tissue, regardless of thickness or greatest dimension; for example, polypoid nasal disease, pigmented or nonpigmented lesions of the oral cavity, pharynx, or larynx |
| T4a | Moderately advanced disease: tumor invades soft tissue, cartilage, bone, or overlying skin |
| T4b | Very advanced disease: tumor invades any of the following deeper structures: brain, dura, skull base, lower cranial nerves (IX, X, XI, XII), masticator space, carotid artery, prevertebral space, or mediastinal structures |
| **N: Regional lymph nodes** | |
| Nx | Regional lymph nodes cannot be assessed |
| N0 | No regional lymph node metastases |
| N1 | Regional lymph node metastasis/metastases present |
| **M: Distant metastasis** | |
| cM0 | No distant metastasis |
| cM1 | Distant metastasis present |
| pM1 | Distant metastasis, microscopically confirmed |
| **Stages** | |
| Stage III | T3 N0 M0 |
| Stage IVA | T4a N0 M0 / T3, T4a N1 M0 |
| Stage IVB | T4b Any N M0 |
| Stage IVC | Any T Any N M1 |

*From* Amin MB, Edge S, Greene F, et al, editors. AJCC Cancer Staging Manual (8th edition). Springer International Publishing: American Joint Commission on Cancer; 2017.

sinonasal mucosal melanoma, radical surgery, including lateral rhinotomy, total rhinectomy, maxillectomy, and craniofacial resection, represents the gold standard. For HNMMs of the oral cavity, adequate resection may involve a marginal or segmental mandibulectomy, and, for mucosal melanomas of the larynx and pharynx, a partial pharyngectomy, partial laryngectomy, or total laryngectomy/pharyngolaryngectomy may be needed to remove the tumor adequately. Careful surgical planning is required to avoid significant morbidity and adverse impact on quality of life that is associated with aggressive surgery, especially in the paranasal sinuses. In this regard, minimally invasive transnasal endoscopic approaches have gained special attention as a way of reducing the likelihood of complications and morbidity while maintaining appropriate oncologic efficacy. Although comparisons between open and endoscopic surgery are all retrospective in nature, all the available literature points to the fact that transnasal resections offers equivalent control rates with lower levels of morbidity.[52]

There is a paucity of evidence that specifically examines the question of contraindications for surgical excision. In general, the inability to achieve negative margins may limit surgical treatment, especially in the context of evidence of intracranial invasion through the dura. In addition, the presence of extensive perineural spread has been associated with poor outcome after surgery and it may influence treatment decisions away from primary surgical management.

There is no established evidence-based consensus regarding the optimal approach to potential regional lymph node disease in patients with HNMMs who present without clinical evidence of lymph node metastasis. From first principles, the options include conservative management and clinical follow-up or surgical intervention in the form of sentinel lymph node biopsy (SLNB) or elective neck dissection (END). The rapid evolution in the field of cutaneous melanoma, as a result of the increasing evidence supporting the use of immunotherapy and targeted treatments in the adjuvant setting, has prompted a change in the role of elective surgery and expanded its use to include procedures that seek to identify patients who may benefit from postoperative systemic therapies. However, in the context on HNMM, most of these considerations do not apply. First, most HNMMs except for oral cavity, arise in mucosal sites that are not readily accessible for direct injection of the dye or radiocolloid that is required for SLNB. In addition, the first echelon draining lymph node group, for instance, the retropharyngeal nodes, may not be amenable to surgical access for sampling. Moreover, the rationale for lymph node sampling that exists for cutaneous melanoma does not apply in the same way, because HNMMs are by definition staged at least as stage III disease and, therefore, eligible for consideration of systemic adjuvant therapy. There is paucity of studies evaluating the efficacy of SLNB in HNMM.[53–55] Therefore, SLNB is not currently recommended in the management of HNMM and its role warrants further investigation.

END is usually not performed for sinonasal mucosal melanomas, because the incidence of nodal disease at the time of presentation is relatively low. However, END has attracted more research in oral mucosal melanomas, where the incidence of regional lymph node metastases is higher, both at initial presentation and during the course of the disease.[56] In this regard, 2 retrospective case series reported no statistically significant higher survival rates in clinically node-negative patients undergoing END (65, 66) with the exception of an association with improved 5-year overall survival (OS) (18% vs 4%, $P = .001$) in patients with nodular oral mucosal melanomas.[57] However, the small cohort of patients involved, the lack of randomization, and the exclusive oral cavity subsite means that one should make guarded recommendations in favor of END in nodular oral melanoma, because the evidence of benefit in this clinical scenario might outweigh the increased morbidity of subjecting patients to such procedure.

## Radiotherapy

The role of radiotherapy as postoperative treatment of HNMM remains unclear. Not surprisingly, radiotherapy has become widely used as part of the treatment algorithm in adjuvant settings with the aim of improving local control. However, no clear data show that postoperative radiotherapy conveys an OS benefit.

Several retrospective studies have reported that the addition of radiotherapy following surgery leads to superior local control rate. In the meta-analysis by Li and colleagues,[58] adjuvant radiation showed a reduction in the risk of local recurrence with a hazard ratio of 0.55 (95% confidence interval between 0.32 and 0.93), which was subsequently confirmed in 2 other systematic reviews.[59] In contrast, other meta-analysis[60] and recent publications[61] have failed to find a significant improvement in local control, probably due to potential bias introduced by the fact that patients at higher risk of local relapse tend to be treated with adjuvant radiotherapy. With regard to OS, none of the historical cohort studies and meta-analyses have demonstrated a significant benefit for patients receiving surgery followed by postoperative radiotherapy. In a contemporaneous data set, Torabi and colleagues[62] demonstrated that although postoperative radiotherapy did not affect OS in nonsinonasal patients, it resulted in improved survival rates for node-negative sinonasal cases. This finding may be a result of limited sample size and partially explained by the fact that regional and distant relapse are more common in primary mucosal melanomas of the oral cavity when compared with sinonasal melanomas.

The understanding of the clinical behavior of HNMM may account for the discrepancy between effectiveness in achieving local control and the lack of effect on OS. Studies of disease recurrence patterns have clearly shown that distant metastases are the main cause of mortality and drive the prognosis of patients with HNMMs. Indeed, local relapses are as low as 20%, whereas distant metastases are observed in up to 80% of the cases, and this is not affected by the use of postoperative radiotherapy.[63] Different publications have reported that around one-half of patients will develop distant relapse at a median interval of 12 months after surgery.[64,65] Thus, precise indications for adjuvant radiation have yet to be defined. Although there is insufficient evidence to identify a particular subgroup of patients who will definitely benefit from adjuvant radiotherapy, there seems to be a higher level of agreement regarding its use in cases with positive or close margins, especially because they represent a negative prognostic marker. The rationale for adjuvant radiotherapy should be to avoid a rapid, symptomatic relapse in the primary site, and it should only be considered in patients in whom benefits in local control are likely to outweigh the risk of series adverse effects.

The optimal radiation dose and fractionation regimens are still undetermined, although conventionally fractionated total doses of more than 54 Gy may improve local control.[39] Mixed results have been reported with regard to the benefit of hypofractionated schedules. A study reported that hypofractionation might improve local control and survival in a series of patients with HNMMs treated with radical intent,[66] whereas other publications have not found that the fractionation schedule exerts any influence on the outcomes.[39,67] Given conventional fractionation could improve the therapeutic ratio by reducing toxicity, especially regarding the optic apparatus, we recommend the use of conventional fractionation schedules. However, one moderately hypofractionated schedule described by Lansu and colleagues,[67] which delivers a total dose of 48 Gy in 20 fractions, could be considered for elderly patients or those with low performance status as a means of limiting the number of visits to the hospital.

New radiation techniques, such as intensity-modulated radiation therapy (IMRT), volumetric-modulated arc therapy (VMAT), tomotherapy, carbon-ion therapy, neutrons, and proton therapy permit the achievement of superior isodose shaping and sharp dose gradients near the targeted values. Photon radiotherapy with IMRT or VMAT remains the standard of care for postoperative radiotherapy. However, an increased number of studies have been recently published about the efficacy and safety of particle therapy (carbon ion, neutrons, and protons) in the treatment of HNMMs, especially used to escalate the radiation dose by sparing uninvolved critical organs. Most of these studies used radiation with radical intent in lymph node-negative patients rather than in the adjuvant setting and, even though none of them is a randomized trial, they reported only a minor improvement in OS rate when compared with historical series of radical surgery and photon-based postoperative radiotherapy. In addition, the reported distant progression-free survival (PFS) does not show marked differences between the 2 treatment modalities and survival remains limited due to early distant metastases, with more than half of the patients showing distant relapse within the first 1 to 3 years after primary treatment.[68–72]

There is limited evidence of the role of radical radiotherapy for unresectable HNMMs. Most of the published series reported a modest local control rate with radiotherapy alone. In studies of definitive radiotherapy with conventional photon techniques, the local control rates are around 60%.[66,73–75] Although the dose and fractionation reported for radical radiotherapy is heterogeneous, a total dose of at least 50 Gy with a moderately hypofractionated schedule has been used in most of the studies.[66,67] Within particle therapy studies, the 5-year local control rate remains around 60%, with exception of Takyasu and colleagues[68] who reported a 5-year local control rate of 82%. However, in that study patients were treated with high-dose concurrent chemotherapy.[68] Moreover, the most recent studies, including a phase 2 study showed a limited PFS of less than 50% at 2 years, due to the high incidence of metastatic disease.[76] Thus, in the uncommon scenario of radical radiotherapy for unresectable HNMMs, particle therapies do not seem to be more effective than conventional photon radiotherapy in improving local control or addressing the dominant clinical problem of distant relapse.

### Adjuvant Systemic Treatment

Considering the high rate of distant failure, and because survival of patients with HNMMs is driven by the early development of distant metastasis, strategies to improve treatment outcome should focus on reducing distant relapse. The arrival of new systemic therapies, such as targeted or immunotherapy, gives a new perspective.

Lian and colleagues[77] published in 2013 the results of the first randomized phase 2 controlled trials addressing the use of adjuvant treatment (observation vs intravenous interferon-α-2b, vs oral temozolomide and intravenous cisplatin) for completely resected mucosal melanoma, including 86 HNMMs. Results showed that median relapse-free survival and estimated median OS were both superior in patients receiving systemic therapy compared with observation. This trial represents the only randomized data in the literature exploring the benefit of adjuvant systemic therapy after resection of HNMM and includes the greatest number of patients with the diagnosis. However, extrapolation of these regimen-specific results is difficult within the current clinical environment because the chemotherapy regimen of temozolomide plus cisplatin has no proven survival benefit in the palliative treatment of metastatic mucosal melanoma. Nevertheless, this study provided the first evidence for a potential role for systemic adjuvant therapy for HNMM following resection with curative intent.

Even though no randomized controlled trial of systemic adjuvant treatment specifically for patients with resected HNMM has been conducted, patients with mucosal melanoma were not excluded from all the more recent randomized, double-blind controlled trials that addressed the use of adjuvant immunotherapy and targeted therapies for advanced melanoma. Indeed, the CheckMate-238 study included 29 patients with mucosal melanoma in a large phase 3 trial of more than 900 patients with resected stage IIIB/C and IV melanoma, randomized to PD-1 inhibitor (nivolumab) compared with anti-CTLA-4 antibody (ipilimumab). The results of this trial showed that adjuvant therapy with nivolumab resulted in significantly better recurrence-free survival than adjuvant therapy with ipilimumab, a longer metastasis-free survival, and a lower rate of grade 3 or 4 adverse events.[78] Although only a small proportion of patients within this study had mucosal melanoma, this randomized study does support a potential role for systemic adjuvant therapy for resected mucosal melanoma and it would not be unreasonable to accept that nivolumab has a role in the adjuvant treatment of HNMM.

None of the other 2 pivotal studies of systemic adjuvant treatment, which have recently changed practice in patients with high-risk cutaneous melanoma, permitted enrollment of patients with mucosal melanoma. These are the Keynote-054[79] and the COMBI-AD studies,[80] both phase

3 double-blind clinical trials that studied the role of adjuvant anti-PD1 (pembrolizumab) and BRAF-directed therapy with BRAF/MEK inhibitors (dabrafenib and trametinib), respectively, for completely resected high-risk stage 3 cutaneous melanoma. The results showed that adjuvant pembrolizumab was associated with significant improvement in recurrence-free survival, and adjuvant dabrafenib/trametinib in patients whose cutaneous melanoma has a targetable BRAF mutation was associated with a 53% reduction in risk of relapse or death. It would not be unreasonable to accept that pembrolizumab may have a role in the adjuvant treatment of HNMM, while acknowledging that this requires both extrapolation of data from the cutaneous melanoma population and assumption of equivalence between nivolumab and pembrolizumab. Moreover, despite the low incidence of activating BRAF V600 mutation in mucosal melanoma, identifying the small subgroup of high-risk patients with resected HNMM and a targetable BRAF mutation is important because they could be considered for adjuvant treatment with BRAF/MEK inhibitors because this will potentially have an impact on their recurrence rate and survival.

## ADVANCED DISEASE AND PALLIATION
### Recurrent Locoregional Disease

Despite radical surgery (with or without adjuvant radiotherapy), a significant proportion of patients with HNMM will suffer from recurrence at local, regional, or distant sites. Even though the poor survival rates for patients with HNMM are mainly attributable to distant metastatic disease, local and/or regional residual and recurrent disease can represent a significant clinical problem. Most data on patterns of treatment failure indicate that isolated local and regional recurrence in the absence of systemic disease is relatively rare and may not in itself have a significant impact on survival.[81]

Local relapse of patients with HNMM is amenable to surgical treatment in only a minority of patients. In this scenario, radical surgery should only be considered a reliable option if complete excision can be achieved, which is often particularly difficult due to the infiltrative pattern of growth of the recurrence. In addition, the rate of surgical complications after a second resection is high and may be unacceptable, especially for those lesions encroaching on vital neurovascular structures of the skull base.[81] Surgical treatment in this context would most likely be debulking surgery with the aim of local disease control or symptom palliation.

There is little evidence regarding the use of radiotherapy to treat local or regional recurrence of HNMMs, especially in the scenario of reirradiation. Despite the fact that relatively high local control (around 79%) has been reported in case series of recurrent HNMM treated with radiotherapy (including reirradiation), survival remains limited by early distant progression.[82] One different approach reported by Kim and colleagues[83] was the use of radiotherapy with concurrent or adjuvant immunotherapy (pembrolizumab). The investigators included 31 patients with mucosal melanoma from different sites, of whom 20 had HNMM. Eleven patients were treated with radiotherapy alone (including 5 primary sites with unresectable disease) to a median dose of 45 Gy, and 12 patients received pembrolizumab concurrently with radiotherapy. Target lesion control was higher in the combination therapy group than in the radiation-alone group (94.1% vs 57.1%). The in-field response rate was similar for both groups, at around 55%. However, once obtained, longer duration of response was achieved in the immunotherapy group than in the radiation-alone group.

In summary, because local and regional recurrence in the absence of systemic disease is relatively rare, considering the high risk of metastatic spread, reflected by the disappointing outcomes when using local therapies alone, and taking into account the recent evidence that immune and targeted therapies offer survival benefit, systemic treatment should be considered the treatment of choice for local and locoregional recurrence in most cases. Local approaches should be limited to palliative options when locoregional control or mitigation of local symptoms are the main goal of therapy.

### Systemic Treatments

#### Immunotherapies
In recent years, the treatment landscape for cutaneous melanoma has changed dramatically with the development of targeted drugs (BRAF and MEK inhibitors) and immune checkpoint inhibitors ([ICIs], anti-CTLA-4, and anti-PD-1 monoclonal antibodies). This change has been reflected in multiple practice-changing phase 3 clinical trials. The relevance of those data to patients with HNMM is largely unknown because most of the landmark studies recruited a population with advanced melanoma dominated by those with cutaneous melanoma and the small numbers of cases with mucosal melanoma make meaningful subgroup analysis difficult.

The most influential publication comprises a reanalysis of pooled data from a series of phase 2 and 3 trials of nivolumab, nivolumab plus ipilimumab, or ipilimumab monotherapy for advanced melanoma[84]; this included around 10% in each cohort with mucosal melanoma, without identification of the site of origin. The key findings were that although there is a clear signal of activity for ICIs, efficacy of each regimen is less than for cutaneous melanoma. Although caution should be exercised in comparing regimens in this analysis, the combination emerged as the most effective, with overall responses rates of 37% and median PFS of 5.9 months. Nivolumab monotherapy resulted in overall response rates of 23% and median PFS of 3 months in the same study. Ipilimumab is the least effective ICI as monotherapy in melanoma generally and resulted in overall response rates of 8% and PFS of 2.7 months in the pooled trials data, with no contradictory study from retrospective data. In advanced melanoma generally, the persuasive data for ICI use is not just based on response rate or median PFS, but the proportion of long-term survivors at 3 and 5 years. However, no such data were provided for mucosal melanoma or HNMM. Another study identified 35 patients with mucosal melanoma treated with anti-PD-1 monotherapy (nivolumab or pembrolizumab). Of the 35 patients, 23% showed an objective response with a median PFS of 3.9 months. Of those with a partial or complete response, the median duration of response was 12.9 months.[85] Finally, a recent publication that included 44 patients with non-surgically-treated, locally advanced and/or metastatic mucosal melanoma (including 18 HNMMs) receiving anti-CTLA-4 and/or anti-PD-1 immunotherapy showed encouraging objective response rates (up to 35% for pembrolizumab) and median PFS (5 months, 95% confidence interval 2.6–33.1 with pembrolizumab).[86]

The observation of lower anti-PD-1 efficacy in mucosal melanoma compared with cutaneous melanoma has prompted research in combination therapies. In this regard, the preliminary results of an open-label phase 1b trial of combination of anti-PD-1 (torapalimumab) with a vascular endothelial growth factor receptor (VEGFR) inhibitor (axitinib) in patients with chemotherapy-naive mucosal melanoma demonstrated promising antitumour activity (response rate of 48.3% and median PFS of 7.5 months).[87]

In conclusion, combination immunotherapy offers an evidence-based treatment option for patients of good performance status with this disease. However, potential toxicity is high, improvement in OS may not be as pronounced as one might expect from the relatively high response rates, and evidence on durability of response in the rare mucosal patient subgroup is lacking. Patients must be counseled on the risks of treatment, and clinicians and patients should be encouraged to consider quality-of-life factors in decision making. For less-fit patients, or those whose preference is to avoid a high risk of potentially serious side effects, anti-PD-1 monotherapy also has evidence to support its efficacy in metastatic mucosal melanoma.

### Targeted therapies

The pivotal phase 3 trials that demonstrated the efficacy of highly selective and high-affinity BRAF inhibitors alone or in combination with MEK inhibition did not include patients diagnosed with mucosal melanoma.[88] However, because up to 15% of patients with HNMM have tumors harboring BRAF mutations, extrapolation of the results from these phase 3 trials seems reasonable. Thus, all patients with mucosal melanoma should be tested for BRAF mutations and, if an activating BRAF mutation is found, then the combination of BRAF and MEK inhibition should be considered.

Around 15% of mucosal melanomas express mutated forms of KIT, and, therefore, tyrosine kinase inhibitors targeting the aberrant protein product have been trialed with some positive results. Two single-arm phase 2 trials have showed clear signal of efficacy for patients with melanoma (including mucosal melanomas) treated with imatinib, with overall response rates of 54% and overall disease control rate of 77% in patients selected for mutated (but not amplified) KIT and response rate of 23.1% in patients with mutated or amplified KIT.[89] Another trial of imatinib in patients with melanoma with KIT mutations or amplifications treated 25 patients. There is also a signal of activity for nilotinib.[90]

NRAS mutations have been found in around 20% of mucosal melanoma and have been associated with a poor prognosis across all melanoma subtypes and represent a potential cause of BRAF and KIT inhibition resistance.[91] Trials are ongoing of drugs targeting the MAPK pathway and the PI3K pathway, which work downstream of NRAS. Indeed, an MEK inhibitor (binimetinib) has been shown to give a response rate of 20% in a phase 2 trial of 30 patients with NRAS-mutated melanoma and a phase 3 trial is ongoing.[92] Trials are also ongoing combining MEK inhibitors with PI3K/AKT inhibitors or CDK4/6 inhibitors.

### Chemotherapy

Until the arrival of ICI and targeted treatments in the last decade, dacarbazine chemotherapy had been the standard of care for metastatic melanoma, with an overall response rate of 13.4%

and a median survival duration ranging from 5.6 to 11 months.[93] Many dacarbazine-based combination regimens have been evaluated in an attempt to improve treatment outcomes. However, all attempts have failed to yield a survival benefit over dacarbazine monotherapy.[94–96]

Combination chemotherapy with carboplatin and paclitaxel has been investigated for both first- and second-line treatment after failure of dacarbazine-based chemotherapy. Two trials of metastatic and advanced melanoma that included patients with mucosal melanoma showed overall response rates of 16% to 18%, median PFS rates of 4.2 months for both studies, and OS rates of 8.6 and 11.3 months. Neither showed advantage for addition of an experimental treatment, bevacizumab or sorafenib.[97,98] A phase 2 randomized trial (abstract only) for advanced mucosal melanoma, without identifying site of origin, also compared carboplatin/paclitaxel chemotherapy with and without bevacizumab, reporting an overall response rate and PFS advantage for the experimental arm supporting progression to phase 3.[99] One Korean study assessed the outcomes of paclitaxel/carboplatin salvage chemotherapy in 32 patients with noncutaneous metastatic melanoma (10 had mucosal melanoma). The median PFS was 2.53 months for all patients, 21.9% achieved partial response, but no significant difference was noted between patients with mucosal and cutaneous metastatic melanoma, suggesting that the effects of chemotherapies are similar in cutaneous melanoma and mucosal melanoma and that, for both subtypes, chemotherapies are usually associated with a poor response rate.[100]

The efficacy of chemotherapy in mucosal melanoma is, thus, poorly defined, and it is now rarely given in melanoma. However, there is renewed interest in the possibility of combining chemotherapy with targeted therapies or immunotherapy, and several trials are underway.

## PROGNOSIS AND FOLLOW-UP

HNMMs are associated with poor clinical outcomes, despite aggressive treatments, with 5-year disease-free survival rates ranging from 0% to 20%; this is because of poor local and distant control and a 5-year OS less than 30% in most series. The median disease-free survival rates are as short as 8 to 12 months in some of the series, and the proportion of patients developing distant metastases ranges from 7% to up to 63%.[10,38,101]

HNMMs behave much more aggressively than their cutaneous counterparts, and their prognostic markers have not been fully elucidated. Clinical stage, surgical margin status, tumor thickness greater than 5 mm, vascular invasion, presence of more than 10 mitotic figures per high-powered field, ulceration, and high Ki67 scores have all been described as independent predictors of outcome.[2,102–104]

Follow-up investigations should be directed at monitoring both local and distant disease relapses, most of which can be expected to occur within the first 2 years after treatment. Early detection of relapse allows treatment with systemic immunotherapies to be started earlier, which may result in a better chance of response. There are no randomized or nonrandomized data on follow-up in the modern era of immunotherapy and targeted treatment to guide recommendations. The recently published United Kingdom national guidelines for HNMMs recommend that following curative treatment or treatment of relapse, all patients should be followed with clinical examination every 6 to 8 weeks; contrast-enhanced cross-sectional imaging of upper aerodigestive tract, neck, thorax, abdomen, and pelvis every 3 weeks; and brain imaging every 6 months during the first year. The frequency of examinations can be reduced to every 3 months during the second and third years and to 6 months from the fourth year, and the cross-sectional imaging of the body and brain can be reduced to every 6 month during years 2 and 3 and every 12 months from the fourth year onward.[105]

## SUMMARY AND FUTURE PERSPECTIVES

Patients diagnosed with HNMM represent a rare subgroup of the melanoma patient population. Although the principles of care are similar, there are critical differences between mucosal and cutaneous melanoma, which must influence future clinical decision making. Although complete surgical excision offers the only prospect of cure, the challenging anatomic sites present a high risk of surgical morbidity and most patients still develop incurable metastatic disease. Endoscopic surgery seems to be suitable when the principles of oncologic surgery with adequate exposure and margins are followed. END should not be performed routinely. There is insufficient evidence to recommend the routine use of postoperative radiotherapy in all patients with HNMM following curative resections, but it may be considered for patients with specific features that denote a particularly high and early risk of local relapse such as positive margins. Systemic treatment with ICI or targeted therapy can offer scope for modifying the course of the disease. Sufficient evidence exists to recommend the use of ICIs or targeted therapies for selected patients with KIT- or BRAF-mutated tumors as adjuvant therapies following curative treatment or for patients with unresectable or metastatic disease. The rarity of the diagnosis will ensure that large-scale mucosal melanoma trials are unlikely ever to be feasible. However, including patients with mucosal melanoma in trials of new agents for the treatment of melanoma will allow us gradually to expand our evidence base and ensure that we identify those regimens that offer more effective anticancer therapies for this small but important patient group.

## CLINICS CARE POINTS

- In the diagnostic process of a patient with suspected HNMM, imaging should precede biopsy and imaging evaluation should include contrast-enhanced cross-sectional CT or MRI of the head and neck region (both should be considered in cases with potential orbital involvement, intracranial and/or perineural disease).

- Systemic staging should include contrast-enhanced CT scan of the thorax, abdomen, and pelvis or full-body PET scan and contrast-enhanced MRI or CT scan of the brain.

- Incisional rather than excisional biopsy is preferred, and molecular analysis of BRAF and C-KIT mutations should be performed routinely.

- Patients with local or locally advanced HNMMs should be reviewed by surgeons who practice in a multidisciplinary team. Surgery should be performed with the aim of obtaining clear margins of excision, and where possible, surgical management should compromise transnasal endoscopic excision (for sinonasal mucosal melanomas). END and SLNB should not be performed routinely.

- Adjuvant radiotherapy may be considered after discussion within a multidisciplinary team for patients with specific features that denote high risk of local recurrence such as T4 sinonasal tumors, close and positive margins, and multifocal primary lesions.

- Adjuvant systemic treatment using ICIs and, where appropriate mutation is present, BRAF-targeted therapies should be considered for all patients.

- In the advanced and metastatic setting, combination immunotherapy (anti-PD1 and anti-CTLA4) should be offered to patients judged as sufficiently fit and willing to accept a high risk of immune-related adverse effects. Otherwise, nivolumab or pembrolizumab monotherapy should be considered if patient is insufficiently fit or does not wish to risk the treated toxicity associated with combination immunotherapy. First-line BRAF or C-KIT-targeted agents should be considered for patients with appropriate mutations, if urgent symptomatic benefit is desired or on failure to immune therapy.

## DISCLOSURE

The authors declare no conflict of interest.

## REFERENCES

1. Chang AE, Karnell LH, Menck HR. The National Cancer Data Base report on cutaneous and noncutaneous melanoma: a summary of 84,836 cases from the past decade. The American College of Surgeons Commission on Cancer and the American Cancer Society. Cancer 1998;83(8):1664–78.
2. Jethanamest D, Vila PM, Sikora AG, et al. Predictors of survival in mucosal melanoma of the head and neck. Ann Surg Oncol 2011;18(10):2748–56.
3. Barrett AW, Raja AM. The immunohistochemical identification of human oral mucosal melanocytes. Arch Oral Biol 1997;42(1):77–81.
4. Natesan SC, Ramakrishnan BP, Krishnapillai R, et al. Biophysiology of oral mucosal melanocytes. J Health Sci Res 2020;10(2):47–51.
5. Gorsky M, Epstein JB. Melanoma arising from the mucosal surfaces of the head and neck. Oral Surg Oral Med Oral Pathol Oral Radiol Endod 1998;86(6):715–9.
6. Iida Y, Salomon MP, Hata K, et al. Predominance of triple wild-type and IGF2R mutations in mucosal melanomas. BMC Cancer 2018;18(1):1054.
7. Holmstrom M, Lund VJ. Malignant melanomas of the nasal cavity after occupational exposure to formaldehyde. Br J Ind Med 1991;48(1):9–11.
8. Hicks MJ, Flaitz CM. Oral mucosal melanoma: epidemiology and pathobiology. Oral Oncol 2000; 36(2):152–69.
9. Nandapalan V, Roland NJ, Helliwell TR, et al. Mucosal melanoma of the head and neck. Clin Otolaryngol Allied Sci 1998;23(2):107–16.
10. Manolidis S, Donald PJ. Malignant mucosal melanoma of the head and neck. Cancer 1997;80(8): 1373–86.
11. Du Z, Lovly CM. Mechanisms of receptor tyrosine kinase activation in cancer. Mol Cancer 2018; 17(1):58.
12. Dhillon AS, Hagan S, Rath O, et al. MAP kinase signalling pathways in cancer. Oncogene 2007; 26(22):3279–90.

13. Carlino MS, Todd JR, Rizos H. Resistance to c-Kit inhibitors in melanoma: insights for future therapies. Oncoscience 2014;1(6):423–6.

14. Phung B, Sun J, Schepsky A, et al. C-KIT signaling depends on microphthalmia-associated transcription factor for effects on cell proliferation. PLoS One 2011;6(8):e24064.

15. Garraway LA, Widlund HR, Rubin MA, et al. Integrative genomic analyses identify MITF as a lineage survival oncogene amplified in malignant melanoma. Nature 2005;436(7047):117–22.

16. Curtin JA, Busam K, Pinkel D, et al. Somatic activation of KIT in distinct subtypes of melanoma. J Clin Oncol 2006;24(26):4340–6.

17. Satzger I, Schaefer T, Kuettler U, et al. Analysis of c-KIT expression and KIT gene mutation in human mucosal melanomas. Br J Cancer 2008;99(12):2065–9.

18. Omholt K, Grafström E, Kanter-Lewensohn L, et al. KIT pathway alterations in mucosal melanomas of the vulva and other sites. Clin Cancer Res 2011;17(12):3933–42.

19. Turri-Zanoni M, Medicina D, Lombardi D, et al. Sinonasal mucosal melanoma: molecular profile and therapeutic implications from a series of 32 cases. Head Neck 2013;35(8):1066–77.

20. Rivera RS, Nagatsuka H, Gunduz M, et al. C-kit protein expression correlated with activating mutations in KIT gene in oral mucosal melanoma. Virchows Arch 2008;452(1):27–32.

21. Newell F, Kong Y, Wilmott JS, et al. Whole-genome landscape of mucosal melanoma reveals diverse drivers and therapeutic targets. Nat Commun 2019;10(1):3163.

22. Dahl C, Guldberg P. The genome and epigenome of malignant melanoma. APMIS 2007;115(10):1161–76.

23. Hayward NK, Wilmott JS, Waddell N, et al. Whole-genome landscapes of major melanoma subtypes. Nature 2017;545(7653):175–80.

24. Edwards RH, Ward MR, Wu H, et al. Absence of BRAF mutations in UV-protected mucosal melanomas. J Med Genet 2004;41(4):270–2.

25. Dumaz N, Jouenne F, Delyon J, et al. Atypical BRAF and NRAS mutations in mucosal melanoma. Cancers (Basel) 2019;11(8):1133.

26. Amit M, Tam S, Abdelmeguid AS, et al. Mutation status among patients with sinonasal mucosal melanoma and its impact on survival. Br J Cancer 2017;116(12):1564–71.

27. Chen F, Zhang Q, Wang Y, et al. KIT, NRAS, BRAF and FMNL2 mutations in oral mucosal melanoma and a systematic review of the literature. Oncol Lett 2018;15(6):9786–92.

28. Chan SH, Chiang J, Ngeow J. CDKN2A germline alterations and the relevance of genotype-phenotype associations in cancer predisposition. Hered Cancer Clin Pract 2021;19(1):21.

29. Bridger AG, Smee D, Baldwin MAR, et al. Experience with mucosal melanoma of the nose and paranasal sinuses. ANZ J Surg 2005;75(4):192–7.

30. Umeda M, Shimada K. Primary malignant melanoma of the oral cavity–its histological classification and treatment. Br J Oral Maxillofac Surg 1994;32(1):39–47.

31. Wenig BM. Laryngeal mucosal malignant melanoma. A clinicopathologic, immunohistochemical, and ultrastructural study of four patients and a review of the literature. Cancer 1995;75(7):1568–77.

32. Prasad ML, Patel SG, Huvos AG, et al. Primary mucosal melanoma of the head and neck: a proposal for microstaging localized, stage I (lymph node-negative) tumors. Cancer 2004;100(8):1657–64.

33. Lourenço SV, Martin Sangüeza A, Sotto MN, et al. Primary oral mucosal melanoma: a series of 35 new cases from South America. Am J Dermatopathol 2009;31(4):323–30.

34. Prasad ML, Jungbluth AA, Iversen K, et al. Expression of melanocytic differentiation markers in malignant melanomas of the oral and sinonasal mucosa. Am J Surg Pathol 2001;25(6):782–7.

35. Thompson LDR, Wieneke JA, Miettinen M. Sinonasal tract and nasopharyngeal melanomas: a clinicopathologic study of 115 cases with a proposed staging system. Am J Surg Pathol 2003;27(5):594–611.

36. Lian B, Cui CL, Zhou L, et al. The natural history and patterns of metastases from mucosal melanoma: an analysis of 706 prospectively-followed patients. Ann Oncol 2017;28(4):868–73.

37. O'Regan K, Breen M, Ramaiya N, et al. Metastatic mucosal melanoma: imaging patterns of metastasis and recurrence. Cancer Imaging 2013;13(4):626–32.

38. Grözinger G, Mann S, Mehra T, et al. Metastatic patterns and metastatic sites in mucosal melanoma: a retrospective study. Eur Radiol 2016;26(6):1826–34.

39. Moreno MA, Roberts DB, Kupferman ME, et al. Mucosal melanoma of the nose and paranasal sinuses, a contemporary experience from the M. D. Anderson Cancer Center. Cancer 2010;116(9):2215–23.

40. McLean N, Tighiouart M, Muller S. Primary mucosal melanoma of the head and neck. Comparison of clinical presentation and histopathologic features of oral and sinonasal melanoma. Oral Oncol 2008;44(11):1039–46.

41. Ascierto PA, Accorona R, Botti G, et al. Mucosal melanoma of the head and neck. Crit Rev Oncol Hematol 2017;112:136–52.

42. Bachar G, Loh KS, O'Sullivan B, et al. Mucosal melanomas of the head and neck: experience of the

Princess Margaret Hospital. Head Neck 2008; 30(10):1325–31.

43. Chan RC-L, Chan JYW, Wei WI. Mucosal melanoma of the head and neck: 32-year experience in a tertiary referral hospital. Laryngoscope 2012; 122(12):2749–53.

44. Kumar V, Vishnoi JR, Kori CG, et al. Primary malignant melanoma of oral cavity: a tertiary care center experience. Natl J Maxillofac Surg 2015;6(2): 167–71.

45. Terada T, Saeki N, Toh K, et al. Primary malignant melanoma of the larynx: a case report and literature review. Auris Nasus Larynx 2007;34(1):105–10.

46. Kim SS, Han MH, Kim JE, et al. Malignant melanoma of the sinonasal cavity: explanation of magnetic resonance signal intensities with histopathologic characteristics. Am J Otolaryngol 2000;21(6): 366–78.

47. Xu Q-G, Fu L-P, Wang Z-C, et al. Characteristic findings of malignant melanoma in the sinonasal cavity on magnetic resonance imaging. Chin Med J (Engl) 2012;125(20):3687–91.

48. Agrawal A, Pantvaidya G, Murthy V, et al. Positron emission tomography in mucosal melanomas of head and neck: results from a South Asian Tertiary Cancer Care Center. World J Nucl Med 2017;16(3): 197–201.

49. Ballantyne AJ. Malignant melanoma of the skin of the head and neck. An analysis of 405 cases. Am J Surg 1970;120(4):425–31.

50. Luna-Ortiz K, Aguilar-Romero M, Villavicencio-Valencia V, et al. Comparative study between two different staging systems (AJCC TNM VS BALLANTYNE'S) for mucosal melanomas of the Head & Neck. Med Oral Patol Oral Cir Bucal 2016;21(4): e425–30.

51. Konuthula N, Khan MN, Parasher A, et al. The presentation and outcomes of mucosal melanoma in 695 patients. Int Forum Allergy Rhinol 2017;7(1): 99–105.

52. Hur K, Zhang P, Yu A, et al. Open versus endoscopic approach for sinonasal melanoma: a systematic review and meta-analysis. Am J Rhinol Allergy 2019;33(2):162–9.

53. Oldenburg MS, Price DL. The utility of sentinel node biopsy for sinonasal melanoma. J Neurol Surg B Skull Base 2017;78(5):425–9.

54. Stárek I, Koranda P, Benes P. Sentinel lymph node biopsy: a new perspective in head and neck mucosal melanoma? Melanoma Res 2006;16(5): 423–7.

55. Prinzen T, Klein M, Hallermann C, et al. Primary head and neck mucosal melanoma: predictors of survival and a case series on sentinel node biopsy. J Craniomaxillofac Surg 2019;47(9):1370–7.

56. Amit M, Tam S, Abdelmeguid AS, et al. Approaches to regional lymph node metastasis in patients with head and neck mucosal melanoma. Cancer 2018;124(3):514–20.

57. Wu Y, Zhong Y, Li C, et al. Neck dissection for oral mucosal melanoma: caution of nodular lesion. Oral Oncol 2014;50(4):319–24.

58. Li W, Yu Y, Wang H, et al. Evaluation of the prognostic impact of postoperative adjuvant radiotherapy on head and neck mucosal melanoma: a meta-analysis. BMC Cancer 2015;15:758.

59. Wushou A, Hou J, Zhao Y-J, et al. Postoperative adjuvant radiotherapy improves loco-regional recurrence of head and neck mucosal melanoma. J Craniomaxillofac Surg 2015;43(4):553–8.

60. Hu R, Yang B-B. Surgery alone versus postoperative radiotherapy for sinonasal malignant melanoma: a meta-analysis. J Laryngol Otol 2018; 132(12):1051–60.

61. Moya-Plana A, Mangin D, Dercle L, et al. Risk-based stratification in head and neck mucosal melanoma. Oral Oncol 2019;97:44–9.

62. Torabi SJ, Benchetrit L, Spock T, et al. Clinically node-negative head and neck mucosal melanoma: an analysis of current treatment guidelines & outcomes. Oral Oncol 2019;92:67–76.

63. Caspers CJI, Dronkers EAC, Monserez D, et al. Adjuvant radiotherapy in sinonasal mucosal melanoma: a retrospective analysis. Clin Otolaryngol 2018;43(2):617–23.

64. Huang S-F, Liao C-T, Kan C-R, et al. Primary mucosal melanoma of the nasal cavity and paranasal sinuses: 12 years of experience. J Otolaryngol 2007;36(2):124–9.

65. Loree TR, Mullins AP, Spellman J, et al. Head and neck mucosal melanoma: a 32-year review. Ear Nose Throat J 1999;78(5):372–5.

66. Wada H, Nemoto K, Ogawa Y, et al. A multi-institutional retrospective analysis of external radiotherapy for mucosal melanoma of the head and neck in Northern Japan. Int J Radiat Oncol Biol Phys 2004;59(2):495–500.

67. Lansu J, Klop WM, Heemsbergen W, et al. Local control in sinonasal malignant melanoma: comparing conventional to hypofractionated radiotherapy. Head Neck 2018;40(1):86–93.

68. Takayasu Y, Kubo N, Shino M, et al. Carbon-ion radiotherapy combined with chemotherapy for head and neck mucosal melanoma: prospective observational study. Cancer Med 2019;8(17): 7227–35.

69. Akimoto T, Zenda S, Nakamura N, et al. A retrospective multi-institutional study of proton beam therapy for head and neck cancer with non-squamous cell histologies. Int J Radiat Oncol Biol Phys 2016;96(2):E337.

70. Demizu Y, Fujii O, Terashima K, et al. Particle therapy for mucosal melanoma of the head and neck: a single-institution retrospective comparison of

proton and carbon ion therapy. Strahlenther Onkol 2014;190(2):186–91.

71. Greenwalt JC, Dagan R, Bryant CM, et al. Proton therapy for sinonasal mucosal melanoma. Int J Radiat Oncol Biol Phys 2015;93(3):E293.

72. Fuji H, Yoshikawa S, Kasami M, et al. High-dose proton beam therapy for sinonasal mucosal malignant melanoma. Radiat Oncol 2014;9(1):162.

73. Douglas CM, Malik T, Swindell R, et al. Mucosal melanoma of the head and neck: radiotherapy or surgery? J Otolaryngol Head Neck Surg 2010; 39(4):385–92.

74. Gilligan D, Slevin NJ. Radical radiotherapy for 28 cases of mucosal melanoma in the nasal cavity and sinuses. BJR 1991;64(768):1147–50.

75. Christopherson K, Malyapa RS, Werning JW, et al. Radiation therapy for mucosal melanoma of the head and neck. Am J Clin Oncol 2015;38(1):87–9.

76. Zenda S, Akimoto T, Mizumoto M, et al. Phase II study of proton beam therapy as a nonsurgical approach for mucosal melanoma of the nasal cavity or para-nasal sinuses. Radiother Oncol 2016; 118(2):267–71.

77. Lian B, Si L, Cui C, et al. Phase II randomized trial comparing high-dose IFN-α2b with temozolomide plus cisplatin as systemic adjuvant therapy for resected mucosal melanoma. Clin Cancer Res 2013;19(16):4488–98.

78. Weber J, Mandala M, Del Vecchio M, et al. Adjuvant nivolumab versus ipilimumab in resected stage III or IV melanoma. N Engl J Med 2017; 377(19):1824–35.

79. Eggermont AMM, Blank CU, Mandala M, et al. Adjuvant pembrolizumab versus placebo in resected stage III melanoma. N Engl J Med 2018; 378(19):1789–801.

80. Long GV, Hauschild A, Santinami M, et al. Adjuvant dabrafenib plus trametinib in stage III BRAF-mutated melanoma. N Engl J Med 2017;377(19): 1813–23.

81. Kaplan DJ, Kim JH, Wang E, et al. Prognostic indicators for salvage surgery of recurrent sinonasal malignancy. Otolaryngol Head Neck Surg 2016; 154(1):104–12.

82. Ladra M, Liao JJ, Parvatheneni U, et al. Fast neutron radiotherapy for locally recurrent and metastatic melanomas of the head and neck. Int J Radiat Oncol Biol Phys 2010;78(3):S470.

83. Kim HJ, Chang JS, Roh MR, et al. Effect of radiotherapy combined with pembrolizumab on local tumor control in mucosal melanoma patients. Front Oncol 2019;9:835.

84. D'Angelo SP, Larkin J, Sosman JA, et al. Efficacy and safety of nivolumab alone or in combination with ipilimumab in patients with mucosal melanoma: a pooled analysis. J Clin Oncol 2017;35(2): 226–35.

85. Shoushtari AN, Munhoz RR, Kuk D, et al. The efficacy of anti-PD-1 agents in acral and mucosal melanoma: PD-1 in acral or mucosal melanoma. Cancer 2016;122(21):3354–62.

86. Moya-Plana A, Herrera Gómez RG, Rossoni C, et al. Evaluation of the efficacy of immunotherapy for non-resectable mucosal melanoma. Cancer Immunol Immunother 2019;68(7):1171–8.

87. Sheng X, Yan X, Chi Z, et al. Axitinib in combination with toripalimab, a humanized immunoglobulin G4 monoclonal antibody against programmed cell death-1, in patients with metastatic mucosal melanoma: an open-label phase IB trial. J Clin Oncol 2019;37(32):2987–99.

88. Robert C, Karaszewska B, Schachter J, et al. Improved overall survival in melanoma with combined dabrafenib and trametinib. N Engl J Med 2015;372(1):30–9.

89. Hodi FS, Corless CL, Giobbie-Hurder A, et al. Imatinib for melanomas harboring mutationally activated or amplified KIT arising on mucosal, acral, and chronically sun-damaged skin. J Clin Oncol 2013;31(26):3182–90.

90. Guo J, Carvajal RD, Dummer R, et al. Efficacy and safety of nilotinib in patients with KIT-mutated metastatic or inoperable melanoma: final results from the global, single-arm, phase II TEAM trial. Ann Oncol 2017;28(6):1380–7.

91. Johnson DB, Puzanov I. Treatment of NRAS-mutant melanoma. Curr Treat Options Oncol 2015;16(4):15.

92. Ascierto PA, Schadendorf D, Berking C, et al. MEK162 for patients with advanced melanoma harbouring NRAS or Val600 BRAF mutations: a non-randomised, open-label phase 2 study. Lancet Oncol 2013;14(3):249–56.

93. Chapman PB, Einhorn LH, Meyers ML, et al. Phase III multicenter randomized trial of the dartmouth regimen versus dacarbazine in patients with metastatic melanoma. J Clin Oncol 1999;17(9):2745–51.

94. Bajetta E, Di Leo A, Zampino MG, et al. Multicenter randomized trial of dacarbazine alone or in combination with two different doses and schedules of interferon alfa-2a in the treatment of advanced melanoma. J Clin Oncol 1994;12(4):806–11.

95. Thomson DB, Adena M, McLeod GR, et al. Interferon-alpha 2a does not improve response or survival when combined with dacarbazine in metastatic malignant melanoma: results of a multi-institutional Australian randomized trial. Melanoma Res 1993;3(2):133–8.

96. Young AM, Marsden J, Goodman A, et al. Prospective randomized comparison of dacarbazine (DTIC) versus DTIC plus interferon-alpha (IFN-alpha) in metastatic melanoma. Clin Oncol (R Coll Radiol) 2001;13(6):458–65.

97. Flaherty KT, Lee SJ, Zhao F, et al. Phase III trial of carboplatin and paclitaxel with or without sorafenib

in metastatic melanoma. J Clin Oncol 2013;31(3): 373–9.

98. Kim KB, Sosman JA, Fruehauf JP, et al. BEAM: a randomized phase II study evaluating the activity of bevacizumab in combination with carboplatin plus paclitaxel in patients with previously untreated advanced melanoma. J Clin Oncol 2012;30(1): 34–41.

99. Yan X, Sheng X, Si L, et al. A randomized phase II study evaluating the activity of bevacizumab in combination with carboplatin plus paclitaxel in patients with previously untreated advanced mucosal melanoma (NCT02023710). J Clin Oncol 2019; 37(15_suppl):9521.

100. Chang W, Lee SJ, Park S, et al. Effect of paclitaxel/carboplatin salvage chemotherapy in noncutaneous versus cutaneous metastatic melanoma. Melanoma Res 2013;23(2):147–51.

101. López F, Rodrigo JP, Cardesa A, et al. Update on primary head and neck mucosal melanoma. Head Neck 2016;38(1):147–55.

102. Patel SG, Prasad ML, Escrig M, et al. Primary mucosal malignant melanoma of the head and neck. Head Neck 2002;24(3):247–57.

103. Shuman AG, Light E, Olsen SH, et al. Mucosal melanoma of the head and neck: predictors of prognosis. Arch Otolaryngol Head Neck Surg 2011; 137(4):331.

104. Kim D-K, Kim DW, Kim SW, et al. Ki67 antigen as a predictive factor for prognosis of sinonasal mucosal melanoma. Clin Exp Otorhinolaryngol 2008;1(4):206–10.

105. Nenclares P, Ap Dafydd D, Bagwan I, et al. Head and neck mucosal melanoma: The United Kingdom national guidelines. Eur J Cancer 2020;138:11–8.

# Adjuvant and Neoadjuvant Therapies in Cutaneous Melanoma

Jay Ponto, MD, DDS, R. Bryan Bell, MD, DDS, FRCS(Ed)*

## KEYWORDS

- Melanoma • Immunotherapy • Adaptive therapy • Head and neck • Metastasis • Systemic therapy
- Malignancy

## KEY POINTS

- Treatment and survival for patients with locally advanced or metastatic melanoma have improved dramatically in the past 10 years.
- Current therapeutic approaches combine immune checkpoint inhibitors with genomically targeted therapies, which are rapidly being incorporated into stage II/III disease, emphasizing enhancing pathologic response at surgery.
- Future directions will involve pretreatment biologic assays to tailor personalized neoadjuvant treatments based upon the immunogenomic profiles.

Melanoma is the most common cause of skin cancer-related death in the United States and cutaneous melanoma is more prevalent in the head and neck than any other anatomic site.[1] The long-term prognosis for patients with metastatic melanoma has traditionally been poor and chemotherapy is not curative. Complete surgical resection for patients with locally advanced disease can be challenging and melanoma is resistant to radiation. In the mid-2000s, there were no effective systemic therapies and virtually all patients with metastatic melanoma died.[2] However, advances made during the last decade in immunotherapy and genomically targeted therapy have transformed the treatment of metastatic melanoma and as of 2021, the 5-year survival for metastatic melanoma is greater than 50%.[3] Most melanomas are diagnosed at an early stage when the lesion is small and surgical excision is curative. However, patients with recurrent metastatic (R/M) disease as well as those with locoregionally advanced disease can be considered for systemic therapy. This review highlights recent advances in the clinical management of R/M and locoregionally advanced melanoma, including changes in staging and the integration of systemic therapy into the neoadjuvant and adjuvant perioperative setting.

## STAGING AND IMMUNOGENOMIC PROFILING

Important changes were made in the 8th edition of the. American Joint Commission on Cancer staging manual that included, for the first time, the use of sentinel lymph node status in final staging.[4] Other important prognostic features of the primary tumor site include depth of invasion, extent of ulceration, and mitotic rate, which are used to estimate the risk of lymph node metastasis. Although mutational analysis, gene expression, and immune profiling are increasingly important in the management of melanoma, the American Joint Commission on Cancer staging manual 8 does not yet include these features in staging. In the future, gene expression signatures and other factors may aid in selecting those patients who will benefit from sentinel lymph node biopsy procedures or adjuvant therapy, but those validation trials are ongoing.

Earle A. Chiles Research Institute in the Robert W. Franz Cancer Center, Providence Cancer Institute, 4805 NE Glisan Street Suite 2N35, Portland, OR 97213, USA
* Corresponding author.
E-mail address: Richard.bell@providence.org

Oral Maxillofacial Surg Clin N Am 34 (2022) 315–324
https://doi.org/10.1016/j.coms.2021.11.010
1042-3699/22/

Comprehensive genomic profiling using next-generation sequencing to guide therapy has already entered the oncology mainstream.[5–7] In melanoma, molecular evaluation reveals it to be among the solid tumors with the highest mutational burden, which is hypothesized to reflect the spectrum of neoantigens that generate an anti-tumor immune response.[8] Tumor mutational burden, as well as programmed death receptor-ligand 1 and IFN-gamma gene signatures are biomarkers that may also predict response to immunotherapy. Although most molecular mutations are not therapeutically relevant, several driver mutations are considered "targetable" in that small molecule kinase inhibitors have been developed or are in the pharmaceutical pipeline as effective genomically targeted therapies. The most important mutation to date is BRAF. BRAF is a serine–threonine kinase in the RAS–RAF–MEK–ERK signaling pathway that was first described in 2002 and is present in approximately 50% of melanomas. RAS mutations occur in about 28% of melanomas.[9] BRAF mutation results in a constitutive activation of MEK and ERK signaling, which suggests that in addition to BRAF inhibition, there may also be a role for blocking these pathways in combination. The contemporary management of stage III or IV melanoma involves reflexive BRAF testing, in addition to selective tumor mutational burden, programmed death receptor-ligand 1, and next-generation sequencing to guide the combination of genomically and immune targeted therapies that are approved by the US Food and Drug Administration (FDA) and clinically available, as well as the plethora of agents in clinical trials.

## BACKGROUND: SYSTEMIC THERAPIES FOR CUTANEOUS METASTATIC MELANOMA

In 1975, the FDA approved the alkylating agent dacarbazine for treatment of patients with unresectable, R/M melanoma. Despite a considerable lack of efficacy in terms of an overall survival benefit, dacarbazine was the treatment of choice for decades and the standard by which other systemic therapies were tested. However, the bar was low; virtually all patients with R/M melanoma who were treated with dacabazine and other chemotherapies died.

Cytokines such as IL-2 and IFN alfa-2b were among the earliest effective therapies for advanced metastatic melanoma. IL-2 is a T-cell growth factor that was first identified in 1976, and its production leads to further T-cell differentiation and activation. The efficacy of high-dose IL-2 for patients with metastatic melanoma was first reported in 1985,[10] leading to FDA approval in 1998.

A subsequent article describing results of IL-2 treatment in 270 patients reported a complete response rate of 6% and a partial response rate of 10%, with a median duration of response greater than 40 months.[11] Remarkably, more than 70% of patients achieving a complete response and approximately 15% of those achieving a partial response remained alive and without recurrence at 15 years, making high-dose IL-2 the first curative immunotherapy regimen for patients with stage IV melanoma. Although a profound cytokine-mediated side effect profile limits wide-spread use of high-dose IL-2 in the current era of immune checkpoint inhibitors, there is substantial evidence to suggest that it can be curative therapy, even in heavily pretreated patients with advanced disease who achieve a complete response.[12–14] It remains an important therapy for patients with R/M disease in some high-volume centers.[14]

## Checkpoint Immunotherapy

Immunotherapy with checkpoint inhibitors that target inhibitory proteins on the surface of T cells, such as cytotoxic T-lymphocyte antigen-4 (CTLA-4) and programmed death 1 (PD-1), have transformed the practice of oncology in general and the treatment of melanoma in particular. CTLA-4 was identified in 1987 by Brunet and colleagues,[15] and in 1995 and 1996 James Allison and colleagues[16,17] discovered its identity as a checkpoint molecule with the potential to halt uncontrolled cell proliferation in preclinical models. CTLA-4 is upregulated on T cells as a result of T-cell receptor engagement by antigen in the lymph nodes and acts as a negative regulator of T-cell activation. Ipilimumab is a human IgG1 monoclonal antibody that binds the CTLA-4 receptor on activated T cells. In a phase III trial published in 2010, ipilimumab-treated patients were found to have a lengthened overall survival by 3.5 months without disease progression compared with a well-studied antineoplastic vaccine using glycoprotein 100.[18] This study led to FDA approval in 2011 for the use of ipilimumab in the treatment of patients with R/M melanoma. Although only 10% of patients responded in the study, the median progression-free survival when treated with ipilimumab was 8 to 12 months. Furthermore, responding patients had a durable benefit: in a study of 1861 patients, ipilimumab was shown to have a 20% survival at 3 years with almost the same 20% still alive at 10 years of follow-up.[19]

PD-1 is another checkpoint receptor on activated T cells and is part of the Ig superfamily, first identified in 1992 by Tasuku Honjo and colleagues.[20] In contrast with CTLA-4, PD-1 is found on a variety of bodily cells including T cells, B cells, natural killer cells, and many peripheral tissue cells. PD-1 promotes T-cell tolerization and is a marker of T-cell exhaustion. The PD-1 protein has an intracellular portion composed of 2 components: an immunoreceptor tyrosine-based inhibitory motif and a immunoreceptor tyrosine-based switch motif.[21] The phosphorylation and activation of the immunoreceptor tyrosine-based inhibitory motif and immunoreceptor tyrosine-based switch motif lead to activation of downstream phosphatases that dephosphorylate T-cell receptor signaling complex, thus inhibiting the activation of T cells. Normally, the activation of T lymphocytes prompts the activation of PD-1, and a successful immune response suppresses PD-1. Blocking antibodies can reverse T-cell exhaustion and enhance antitumor activity in some patients and have shown even greater clinical efficacy than anti–CTLA-4.

The first evidence of efficacy for PD-1 blockade was with the fully human monoclonal antibody nivolumab. Results of a phase I dose escalation trial were published in 2012, which demonstrated a 37.5% objective response rate in multiple tumor types.[22] The anti–PD-1 antibody pembrolizumab entered clinical testing in April 2011 and, with the encouraging clinical data from nivolumab, pembrolizumab's clinical development focused on patients with metastatic melanoma, resulting in the largest phase I trial ever conducted in oncology, eventually enrolling 1235 patients with a similar response rate and durable tumor remission.[23]

When compared with ipilimumab in phase III trials treating advanced melanoma, both nivolumab and pembrolizumab have shown better efficacy and decreased side effects.[24,25] In the Checkmate-67 clinical trial, patients treated with nivolumab plus ipilimumab had a median overall survival of more than 60 months compared with 39.9 months and 19.9 months for nivolumab and ipilimumab monotherapies, respectively. However, the combination versus nivolumab alone had overall survival of 52 versus 44 months, which was not statistically different. The overall survival of ipilimumab alone was 29 months. Ipilimumab combined with nivolumab has been associated with a 53% response rate and is now the standard of care for immunotherapy in most patients with advanced melanoma.[26–28]

## Genomically Targeted Therapy: BRAF and MEK Inhibitors

The mitogen-activated protein kinase pathway is an intracellular molecular cascade that regulates cellular proliferation, mitosis, gene expression, and a myriad of other cellular functions. Once the extracellular epidermal growth factor binds to its receptor within the cell, RAS is activated, which in turn activates BRAF.[9] BRAF activation then leads to the phosphorylation of other molecules, including MEK, which is discussed elsewhere in this article. This phosphorylation sequence eventually leads to nuclear transcription factor activation and increased cellular proliferation. BRAF mutations are present in 50% of melanomas, the most common subtype of which is V600E mutation, which has been identified in more than 70% of BRAF mutations overall.[29]

Targeted therapies are usually small molecule drugs capable of binding to the mutated gene sequences in tumor cells, which leads to inhibited cellular proliferation. Small molecules currently being used to inhibit BRAF include vemurafenib, dabrafenib, and encorafenib. In 2011, Vemurafenib became the first BRAF inhibitor to be approved by the FDA for the treatment of advanced melanoma, based on a 48% response rate and a 63% reduction in the risk of death compared with dacarbazine chemotherapy.[30] Although tumor regression after vemurafenib therapy is usually brisk and clinically meaningful, progression-free survival is only 5.3 months, which is typical of the resistance to mitogen-activated protein kinase pathway inhibitors that occurs when they are given by themselves (monotherapy); virtually all patients develop resistance. Other BRAF inhibitors, such as dabrafenib and encorafenib, generate similar response rates and resistance profiles.[31,32]

As mentioned elsewhere in this article, MEK is a protein kinase that is activated via phosphorylation by BRAF in the mitogen-activated protein kinase pathway. Once activated, MEK stimulates ERK, furthering a signaling cascade that leads to transcription factor activation and increased cellular proliferation. Trametinib was the first FDA-approved MEK inhibitor, approved for monotherapy in 2013 after demonstrating improved overall survival, response rates, and progression-free survival in patients treated with trametinib versus traditional cytotoxic chemotherapy.[33] It turns out that MEK inhibitors work well in tumors with BRAF mutations, but unfortunately MEK inhibitors are less effective than BRAF inhibitors when used as monotherapy. However, MEK inhibitors, including cobimetinib, pimasertib, selumetinib, binimetinib, and trametinib, have been tested in combination with BRAF inhibitors, which have been shown to be more efficacious than BRAF inhibitors alone and show fewer side effects, with response rated in excess of 60% and complete response rates between 10% and 18%.[34,35] Therefore, this duo has become the standard of care in the treatment of BRAF-positive metastatic melanomas because more than 90% of BRAF-mutated melanomas seem to have an initial response to this dual therapy.[34,36]

BRAF inhibitors have been not been compared side by side, but have been compared across different trials when paired with corresponding MEK inhibitors. Encorafenib/binimetinib showed a longer overall survival rate (33.6 months in the COLUMBUS trial)[37] compared with vemurafenib/cobimetinib (22.3 months in the coBRIM trial)[38] and dabrafenib/trametinib (25.6 months in the COMBI-v trial).[39]

## ADJUVANT THERAPY

IFN alpha-2b was the first agent to significantly affect the relapse-free survival of patients with a high risk of relapse after surgical resection.[40] Based on studies that demonstrated a 17% lower relapse risk compared with untreated controls, it was first approved by the FDA in 1995 and was for many years a standard treatment option for patients with stage IIb or III resected melanoma. In 2011, a form of interferon conjugated with polyethylene glycol used as a protective agent to delay molecular breakdown and increase the drug's half-life was FDA approved. This new pegylated interferon was approved after a single phase III, open-label, randomized, multicenter trial showed no survival difference, but did demonstrate a relapse-free-survival difference of 34.8 months versus 25.5 months in the pegylated interferon and observation arms, respectively.[41]

In contrast, ipilimumab was the first agent to demonstrate an improved progression-free survival (40.8%) and overall survival (65.4%) benefit that was durable in responding patients, compared with placebo (30.3% and 54.4%, respectively) in the adjuvant setting (**Table 1**).[36,42] Ipilimumab at 3 mg or 10 mg also outperformed IFN alf-2b in a phase III trial for patients with stage IIIB and IIIC disease by generating an overall 5-year survival rate of 70% to 72% in the ipilimumab arm compared with 63% in the interferon arm.[43] However, in subsequent phase III clinical trials, both nivolumab (CheckMate 238)[44] and pembrolizumab (KEYNOTE-054)[45] have shown improved efficacy and a decrease in toxicity compared with ipilimumab, making these agents the current standard of care for adjuvant therapy in patients with resected stage III BRAF wild-type melanomas. In Checkmate 238, treatment with nivolumab resulted in 70.5% relapse-free survival compared with 60.8% relapse-free survival for ipilimumab. For patients with surgically resected stage IV melanomas, the combination of ipilimumab and nivolumab seems to be most favorable.[46]

Targeted therapies are also being studied in the adjuvant setting. In a randomized, double-blind study of patients with stage III melanoma, the combination of dabrafenib plus trametinib decreased the probability of recurrence and death by 53% and 42%, respectively, compared with placebo.[47] Furthermore, 52% of patients in the combined therapy group remained disease free at 5 years compared with 36% of those in the placebo group.[48] Since this pivotal study, combined BRAF and MEK inhibition has become the standard of care in the adjuvant setting for patients with stage III BRAF-mutant melanoma.

The combination of immune checkpoint inhibitors with genomically targeted therapies in the adjuvant setting is an approach under investigation and seems to have added benefit in patients with resected stage IIIB, stage IIIC, and stage IV melanomas. Comparisons of various combinations are unlikely to occur, but these agents remain treatment options at the discretion of the treating physician. There is an ongoing phase III trial comparing immune checkpoint inhibition with surveillance in patients with stage IIB or IIC disease whose tumors display deep invasion or ulceration (NCT04099251), which could result in a new standard of care for these patients in the future. Most recently, on December 3, 2021, the FDA approved pembrolizumab for the adjuvant treatment of adult and pediatric ($\geq$12 years of age) patients with stage IIB or IIC melanoma following complete resection. Efficacy was evaluated in KEYNOTE-716 (NCT03553836), a multicenter, randomized (1:1), double-blind, placebo-controlled trial in patients with completely resected stage IIB or IIC melanoma, which demonstrated a statistically significant improvement in RFS for patients randomized to the pembrolizumab arm compared with placebo, with a hazard ratio of 0.65 (95% CI: 0.46, 0.92; p=0.0132). The median RFS was not reached in either arm.[49]

## NEOADJVUANT THERAPY

There is preclinical evidence that administering neoadjuvant immunotherapy before surgery is superior to that of adjuvant therapy.[50] Recently, Huang and colleagues[51] demonstrated that a complete pathologic response or major pathologic response (defined as <10% viable tumor cells) after a single dose of anti–PD-1 was associated with improved disease-free survival in patients with high-risk resectable stage III/IV melanoma. These pathologic responses were associated with

**Table 1**
Adjuvant therapies according to clinical trial

| | EORTC 18071 | ECOG 1609 | CheckMate 238 | Eortc 1325 | COMBI-AD |
|---|---|---|---|---|---|
| Eligible stages | Stage IIIA[a], B, and C | Stage IIIB and C; M1a and b | Stage IIIB and C, IV | Stage IIIA[a], B, and C | Stage IIIA[a], B, and C |
| Study groups (number of patients) | Ipilimumab (475) vs placebo (476) | Ipilimumab 3 mg (523) vs ipilimumab 10 mg (511) vs interferon (636) | Nivolumab (453) vs ipilimumab (453) | Pembrolizumab (514) vs placebo (505) | Dabrafenib + trametinib (435) vs dual placebo (432) |
| Relapse-free survival | 40.8% vs 30.3% at 5 y | Median, 4.5 y vs 3.9 y vs 2.5 y | 70.5% vs 60.8% at 12 mo | 63.7% vs 44.1% at 3 y | 52% vs 36% at 5 y |
| Overall survival | 65.4% vs 54.4% at 5 y | 72% vs 70% vs 63% at 5 y | Not reported | Not reported | 86% vs 77% at 3 y |

[a] In stage IIIA, nodal metastasis had to be more than 1 mm in the longest dimension.
*Adapted from* Curti, BD, Faries, MB. Recent Advances in the Treatment of Melanoma. N Engl J Med 2021; 384:2229-40.

**Table 2**
Neoadjuvant therapies according to clinical trial

| | Amaria et al | OpACIN | NeoCombi | Huang et al | OpACIN-Neo |
|---|---|---|---|---|---|
| Eligible clinical stages | Stage III or IV (BRAF-mutated) | Stage III or IV | Stage III | Stage III (BRAF-mutated) | Stage III or IV | Stage III |
| Preoperative treatment (number of patients) | Dabrafenib + trametinib for 8 wk (14) vs none (7) | Nivolumab 3 mg (12) vs ipilimumab 3 mg + nivolumab 1 mg (11) for 12 wk | Ipilimumab 3 mg + nivolumab 1 mg for 6 wk (10) vs none (10) | Dabrafenib + trametinib for 12 wk (35) | Single-dose pembrolizumab, resection at 3 wk (30) | 2 courses ipilimumab 3 mg + nivolumab 1 mg (30) vs 2 COURSES Ipilimumab 1 mg + nivolumab 3 mg (30) vs 2 courses ipilimumab 3 mg followed by 2 courses nivolumab 3 mg (26)[a] |
| Postoperative treatment | Dabrafenib + trametinib vs observation until recurrence | Nivolumab 3 mg vs ipilimumab 3 mg + nivolumab 1 mg for 24 wk | Ipilimumab 3 mg + nivolumab 1 mg for 6 wk vs for 12 wk | Dabrafenib + trametinib for 40 wk | Pembrolizumab for 1 y | None |
| Relapse-free survival | Median, 19.7 mo vs 2.9 mo | Ipilimumab + nivolumab, 90% at 14.9 mo | No relapse in the neoadjuvant group at 25.6 mo | Median, 23 mo | 100% among patients with near (30% of patients) or complete pathologic response | Not mature (no deaths from melanoma in patients with pathologic response) |

[a] Two courses of therapy (1 course every 3 weeks) were administered for each treatment group.

*Adapted from* Curti, BD, Faries, MB. Recent Advances in the Treatment of Melanoma. N Engl J Med 2021; 384:2229-40.

accumulation of tumor-infiltrating lymphocytes that, likewise, were associated with clinical benefit. Thus, studies to assess complete pathologic response as an end point in neoadjuvant studies with immunotherapies are ongoing. Furthermore, immunotherapy in the neoadjuvant setting is of considerable biologic interest, because tumor, metastatic, and draining lymph nodes are readily available before and after treatment, which provides a source of tissue for multi-omic interrogation.[52]

Both targeted therapies and immunotherapies have been shown to produce a complete pathologic response rate of approximately 30% in neoadjuvant setting (**Table 2**).[53–56] Neoadjuvant BRAF plus MEK inhibition before surgery resulted in a significantly longer event-free survival rate than surgery alone in a recent phase II trial.[57] The combination of ipilimumab and nivolumab increases the complete pathologic response rate to 45%, but at a cost of increasing treatment-related grade 3 toxicities of 73%.[54] Subsequent studies suggested an improved safety profile if ipilimumab is given once and nivolumab is given 3 times before surgery.[58] The OpACIN-neo (Optimal Neoadjuvant Combination Scheme of Ipilimumab and Nivolumab) trial used a modified regimen of a lower dose ipilimumab (1 mg/kg) and only 2 doses of nivolumab (3 mg/kg), which resulted in a 57% response rate with modest toxicity.[58] In this trial, the pathologic response rate was 100% in patients with high tumor mutational burden and high IFN-$\gamma$ score,[59] and the 2-year estimated relapse-free survival was 97% for patients achieving a pathologic response. In contrast, only 36% of nonresponders had a relapse-free survival at 2 years.

The role of pathologic response rate and its impact on clinical benefit was recently also evaluated for 6 trials where neoadjuvant treatment was given to melanoma patients (n = 192).[60] The majority of the patients received immunotherapy (n = 141), and 51 patients received targeted therapies. Importantly, of the 40% of patients who had a complete pathologic response, 47% were associated with targeted therapies and 33% with immunotherapy. Patients receiving a combination of ipilimumab and nivolumab demonstrated a 43% complete pathologic response rate. Similar to breast cancer, the complete pathologic response rate translated to an overall survival benefit assessed at 2 years: patients with a complete pathologic response to immunotherapy were virtually all alive, with a relapse-free survival of 96%. By contrast, patients treated with targeted agents had an overall survival rate of 91% and relapse-free survival of 79%.[60]

Of considerable interest to surgeons is the question of whether the extent of surgery can be decreased after a treatment response with either immunotherapy or targeted therapy. Ongoing trials, including the Personalized Response-Driven Adjuvant Therapy after OpACIN (PRADO) trial, are attempting to answer this question.

As with adjuvant therapy, no randomized trials comparing targeted therapy to immunotherapy in the neoadjuvant setting have been performed. However, the extremely high rate of disease control and strong association with improved survival observed after a major response to checkpoint blockade has fostered considerable enthusiasm for this approach.

## Future Directions

Given the large number of immunotherapies and targeted agents in the developmental pipeline, improved predictive biomarkers are urgently needed to tailor therapy moving forward. One such platform involves the use of patient-derived tumor explants and the testing of novel drug combinations ex vivo.[61,62] In addition, novel combinations of checkpoint inhibitors with targeted agents and other immune modulators in the neoadjuvant or adjuvant setting are of interest, including tumor necrosis factor[63] and the Toll-like agonistic compounds. Some of the Toll-like agonists seem to increase IFN-$\gamma$ production in the absence of T-cell recruitment[64,65] and can be combined with other therapies as T-cell primers with agents designed to recruit T cells to the tumor. The future will involve personalized therapy based on their individual tumor tissue expression profile with an approach that matches an individual patient to novel or standard treatments in combination with surgery to enhance the complete pathologic response rate in neoadjuvant setting.

## CLINICS CARE POINTS

1. Owing to recent advances in immunotherapy over the last 2 decades, the 5-year survival rate for malignant melanoma is now more than 50%.

2. Molecular evaluation of melanomas has shown melanoma to be among solid tumors with the highest mutational burden, which is hypothesized to reflect the spectrum of neoantigens that can generate an antitumor immune response.

3. Checkpoint inhibitor immunotherapy began with ipilimumab in 2011. Although

only a small percentage of patients responded, the response was shown to be meaningful and long-term.

4. MEK inhibitors in combination with BRAF inhibitors is the standard of care in the treatment of BRAF positive metastatic melanomas.

5. Nivolumab and pembrolizumab treatment is the current standard of care for adjuvant therapy in patients with resected stage III BRAF wild-type melanomas.

6. As of December 2021, the FDA has granted approval to pembrolizumab (Keytruda) for the adjuvant treatment of both adult and pediatric patients aged 12 years and older with stage IIB or IIC melanoma following complete resection.

7. The combination of ipilimumab and nivolumab is most favorable treatment for patients with surgically resected stage IV melanomas.

8. In comparing combinations of BRAF and MEK inhibitors, encorafenib/binimetinib showed a longer overall survival rate compared with vemurafenib/cobimetinib and dabrafenib/trametinib.

9. Combined BRAF and MEK inhibition has become the standard of care in the adjuvant setting for patients with stage III BRAF-mutant melanoma.

10. No randomized trials comparing targeted therapy with immunotherapy in the adjuvant or neoadjuvant setting have been performed; however, the use of checkpoint inhibitors with genomically targeted therapy has shown added benefit with both these treatment modalities.

11. The future will involve personalized therapy based on an individual tumor tissue expression profiles with an approach that matches an individual patient to novel or standard treatments in combination with surgery to enhance the pathologic complete response rate in neoadjuvant setting.

## REFERENCES

1. Henley SJ, Ward EM, Scott S, et al. Annual report to the nation on the status of cancer, part I: national cancer statistics. Cancer 2020;126:2225–49.

2. Korn EL, Liu PY, Lee SJ, et al. Meta-analysis of phase II cooperative group trials in metastatic stage IV melanoma to determine progression-free and overall survival benchmarks for future phase II trials. J Clin Oncol 2008;26:527–34.

3. Curti BD, Faries MB. Recent Advances in the Treatment of Melanoma. N Engl J Med 2021;384:2229–40.

4. Gershenwald JE, Scolyer RA, Hess KR, et al. Melanoma staging: evidence-based changes in the American Joint Committee on Cancer eighth edition cancer staging manual. CA Cancer J Clin 2017;67:472–92.

5. Marchetti MA, Coit DG, Dusza SW, et al. Performance of gene expression profile tests for prognosis in patients with localized cutaneous melanoma: a systematic review and meta-analysis. JAMA Dermatol 2020;156:953–62.

6. Vetto JT, Hsueh EC, Gastman BR, et al. Guidance of sentinel lymph node biopsy decisions in patients with T1-T2 melanoma using gene expression profiling. Future Oncol 2019;15:1207–17.

7. Eggermont AMM, Bellomo D, Arias-Mejias SM, et al. Identification of stage I/IIA melanoma patients at high risk for disease relapse using a clinicopathologic and gene expression model. Eur J Cancer 2020;140:11–8.

8. Jiang J, Ding Y, Wu M, et al. Integrated genomic analysis identifies a genetic mutation model predicting response to immune checkpoint inhibitors in melanoma. Cancer Med 2020;9:8498–518.

9. Davies H, Bignell GR, Cox C, et al. Mutations of the BRAF gene in human cancer. Nature 2002;417:949–54.

10. Rosenberg SA, Lotze MT, Muul LM, et al. Observations on the systemic administration of autologous lymphokine-activated killer cells and recombinant interleukin-2 to patients with metastatic cancer. N Engl J Med 1985;313:1485–92.

11. Atkins MB, Lotze MT, Dutcher JP, et al. High-dose recombinant interleukin 2 therapy for patients with metastatic melanoma: analysis of 270 patients treated between 1985 and 1993. J Clin Oncol 1999;17:2105–16.

12. Clark JI, Curti B, Davis EJ, et al. Long-term progression-free survival of patients with metastatic melanoma or renal cell carcinoma following high-dose interleukin-2. J Investig Med. 2021 Feb 4;69(4):888–92.

13. Curti B, Crittenden M, Seung SK, et al. Randomized phase II study of stereotactic body radiotherapy and interleukin-2 versus interleukin-2 in patients with metastatic melanoma. J Immunother Cancer 2020;8.

14. Payne R, Glenn L, Hoen H, et al. Durable responses and reversible toxicity of high-dose interleukin-2 treatment of melanoma and renal cancer in a Community Hospital Biotherapy Program. J Immunother Cancer 2014;2:13.

15. Brunet JF, Denizot F, Luciani MF, et al. A new member of the immunoglobulin superfamily–CTLA-4. Nature 1987;328:267–70.

16. Leach DR, Krummel MF, Allison JP. Enhancement of antitumor immunity by CTLA-4 blockade. Science 1996;271:1734–6.

17. Krummel MF, Allison JP. CD28 and CTLA-4 have opposing effects on the response of T cells to stimulation. J Exp Med 1995;182:459–65.

18. Hodi FS, O'Day SJ, McDermott DF, et al. Improved survival with ipilimumab in patients with metastatic melanoma. N Engl J Med 2010;363:711–23.

19. Schadendorf D, Hodi FS, Robert C, et al. Pooled Analysis of Long-Term Survival Data From Phase II and Phase III Trials of Ipilimumab in Unresectable or Metastatic Melanoma. J Clin Oncol 2015;33:1889–94.

20. Ishida Y, Agata Y, Shibahara K, et al. Induced expression of PD-1, a novel member of the immunoglobulin gene superfamily, upon programmed cell death. EMBO J 1992;11:3887–95.

21. Nishimura H, Nose M, Hiai H, et al. Development of lupus-like autoimmune diseases by disruption of the PD-1 gene encoding an ITIM motif-carrying immunoreceptor. Immunity 1999;11:141–51.

22. Topalian SL, Hodi FS, Brahmer JR, et al. Safety, activity, and immune correlates of anti-PD-1 antibody in cancer. N Engl J Med 2012;366:2443–54.

23. Garon EB, Rizvi NA, Hui R, et al. Pembrolizumab for the treatment of non-small-cell lung cancer. N Engl J Med 2015;372:2018–28.

24. Hodi FS, Chiarion-Sileni V, Gonzalez R, et al. Nivolumab plus ipilimumab or nivolumab alone versus ipilimumab alone in advanced melanoma (CheckMate 067): 4-year outcomes of a multicentre, randomised, phase 3 trial. Lancet Oncol 2018;19:1480–92.

25. Schachter J, Ribas A, Long GV, et al. Pembrolizumab versus ipilimumab for advanced melanoma: final overall survival results of a multicentre, randomised, open-label phase 3 study (KEYNOTE-006). Lancet 2017;390:1853–62.

26. Wolchok JD, Kluger H, Callahan MK, et al. Nivolumab plus ipilimumab in advanced melanoma. N Engl J Med 2013;369:122–33.

27. Callahan MK, Kluger H, Postow MA, et al. Nivolumab plus ipilimumab in patients with advanced melanoma: updated survival, response, and safety data in a phase I dose-escalation study. J Clin Oncol 2018;36:391–8.

28. Postow MA, Chesney J, Pavlick AC, et al. Nivolumab and ipilimumab versus ipilimumab in untreated melanoma. N Engl J Med 2015;372:2006–17.

29. melanoma. TCGANGcoc, 1681-1696. C.

30. Chapman PB, Hauschild A, Robert C, et al. Improved survival with vemurafenib in melanoma with BRAF V600E mutation. N Engl J Med 2011;364:2507–16.

31. Long GV, Stroyakovskiy D, Gogas H, et al. Combined BRAF and MEK inhibition versus BRAF inhibition alone in melanoma. N Engl J Med 2014;371:1877–88.

32. Long GV, Flaherty KT, Stroyakovskiy D, et al. Dabrafenib plus trametinib versus dabrafenib monotherapy in patients with metastatic BRAF V600E/K-mutant melanoma: long-term survival and safety analysis of a phase 3 study. Ann Oncol 2017;28:1631–9.

33. Falchook GS, Lewis KD, Infante JR, et al. Activity of the oral MEK inhibitor trametinib in patients with advanced melanoma: a phase 1 dose-escalation trial. Lancet Oncol 2012;13:782–9.

34. Robert C, Grob JJ, Stroyakovskiy D, et al. Five-Year outcomes with dabrafenib plus trametinib in metastatic melanoma. N Engl J Med 2019;381:626–36.

35. Dummer R, Ascierto PA, Gogas HJ, et al. Overall survival in patients with BRAF-mutant melanoma receiving encorafenib plus binimetinib versus vemurafenib or encorafenib (COLUMBUS): a multicentre, open-label, randomised, phase 3 trial. Lancet Oncol 2018;19:1315–27.

36. Eggermont AMM, Chiarion-Sileni V, Grob JJ, et al. Adjuvant ipilimumab versus placebo after complete resection of stage III melanoma: long-term follow-up results of the European Organisation for Research and Treatment of Cancer 18071 double-blind phase 3 randomised trial. Eur J Cancer 2019;119:1–10.

37. Dummer R, Ascierto PA, Gogas HJ, et al. Encorafenib plus binimetinib versus vemurafenib or encorafenib in patients with BRAF-mutant melanoma (COLUMBUS): a multicentre, open-label, randomised phase 3 trial. Lancet Oncol 2018;19:603–15.

38. Ascierto PA, McArthur GA, Dreno B, et al. Cobimetinib combined with vemurafenib in advanced BRAF(V600)-mutant melanoma (coBRIM): updated efficacy results from a randomised, double-blind, phase 3 trial. Lancet Oncol 2016;17:1248–60.

39. Hamid O, Cowey CL, Offner M, et al. Efficacy, Safety, and Tolerability of Approved Combination BRAF and MEK Inhibitor Regimens for BRAF-Mutant Melanoma. Cancers (Basel) 2019;11.

40. Kirkwood JM, Ibrahim JG, Sondak VK, et al. High- and low-dose interferon alfa-2b in high-risk melanoma: first analysis of intergroup trial E1690/S9111/C9190. J Clin Oncol 2000;18:2444–58.

41. Eggermont AM, Suciu S, Santinami M, et al. Adjuvant therapy with pegylated interferon alfa-2b versus observation alone in resected stage III melanoma: final results of EORTC 18991, a randomised phase III trial. Lancet 2008;372:117–26.

42. Eggermont AM, Chiarion-Sileni V, Grob JJ, et al. Prolonged survival in stage III melanoma with ipilimumab adjuvant therapy. N Engl J Med 2016;375:1845–55.

43. Tarhini AA, Lee SJ, Hodi FS, et al. Phase III study of adjuvant ipilimumab (3 or 10 mg/kg) versus high-dose interferon Alfa-2b for resected high-risk melanoma: North American Intergroup E1609. J Clin Oncol 2020;38:567–75.

44. Ascierto PA, Del Vecchio M, Mandala M, et al. Adjuvant nivolumab versus ipilimumab in resected stage IIIB-C and stage IV melanoma (CheckMate 238): 4-year results from a multicentre, double-blind, randomised, controlled, phase 3 trial. Lancet Oncol 2020; 21:1465–77.

45. Eggermont AMM, Blank CU, Mandala M, et al. Adjuvant pembrolizumab versus placebo in resected stage III melanoma (EORTC 1325-MG/KEYNOTE-054): distant metastasis-free survival results from a double-blind, randomised, controlled, phase 3 trial. Lancet Oncol 2021;22:643–54.

46. Zimmer L, Livingstone E, Hassel JC, et al. Adjuvant nivolumab plus ipilimumab or nivolumab monotherapy versus placebo in patients with resected stage IV melanoma with no evidence of disease (IMMUNED): a randomised, double-blind, placebo-controlled, phase 2 trial. Lancet 2020;395:1558–68.

47. Long GV, Hauschild A, Santinami M, et al. Adjuvant Dabrafenib plus Trametinib in Stage III BRAF-Mutated Melanoma. N Engl J Med 2017;377: 1813–23.

48. Dummer R, Hauschild A, Santinami M, et al. Five-Year Analysis of Adjuvant Dabrafenib plus Trametinib in Stage III Melanoma. N Engl J Med 2020; 383:1139–48.

49. Luke JJ, Rutkowski P, Querirolo P, et al. Pembrolizumab versus placebo after complete resection of high-risk stage II melanoma: efficacy and safety results from the KEYNOTE-716 double-blind phase III trial. Ann Oncol (ESMO Congress Abstracts) 2021; 32(suppl 5. Abstract LBA3_PR). https://doi.org/10.1016/annonc/annonc741.

50. Liu J, Blake SJ, Yong MC, et al. Improved efficacy of neoadjuvant compared to adjuvant immunotherapy to eradicate metastatic disease. Cancer Discov 2016;6:1382–99.

51. Huang AC, Orlowski RJ, Xu X, et al. A single dose of neoadjuvant PD-1 blockade predicts clinical outcomes in resectable melanoma. Nat Med 2019;25: 454–61.

52. Maio M, Blank C, Necchi A, et al. Neoadjuvant immunotherapy is reshaping cancer management across multiple tumour types: the future is now. Eur J Cancer 2021;152:155–64.

53. Sloot S, Zager JS, Kudchadkar RR, et al. BRAF inhibition for advanced locoregional BRAF V600E mutant melanoma: a potential neoadjuvant strategy. Melanoma Res 2016;26:83–7.

54. Amaria RN, Reddy SM, Tawbi HA, et al. Neoadjuvant immune checkpoint blockade in high-risk resectable melanoma. Nat Med 2018;24:1649–54.

55. Blank CU, Rozeman EA, Fanchi LF, et al. Neoadjuvant versus adjuvant ipilimumab plus nivolumab in macroscopic stage III melanoma. Nat Med 2018; 24:1655–61.

56. Sun J, Kirichenko DA, Zager JS, et al. The emergence of neoadjuvant therapy in advanced melanoma. Melanoma Manag 2019;6:MMT27.

57. Amaria RN, Prieto PA, Tetzlaff MT, et al. Neoadjuvant plus adjuvant dabrafenib and trametinib versus standard of care in patients with high-risk, surgically resectable melanoma: a single-centre, open-label, randomised, phase 2 trial. Lancet Oncol 2018;19: 181–93.

58. Rozeman EA, Menzies AM, van Akkooi ACJ, et al. Identification of the optimal combination dosing schedule of neoadjuvant ipilimumab plus nivolumab in macroscopic stage III melanoma (OpACIN-neo): a multicentre, phase 2, randomised, controlled trial. Lancet Oncol 2019;20:948–60.

59. Rozeman EA, Hoefsmit EP, Reijers ILM, et al. Survival and biomarker analyses from the OpACIN-neo and OpACIN neoadjuvant immunotherapy trials in stage III melanoma. Nat Med 2021;27:256–63.

60. Menzies AM, Amaria RN, Rozeman EA, et al. Pathological response and survival with neoadjuvant therapy in melanoma: a pooled analysis from the International Neoadjuvant Melanoma Consortium (INMC). Nat Med 2021;27:301–9.

61. Voabil P, de Bruijn M, Roelofsen LM, et al. An ex vivo tumor fragment platform to dissect response to PD-1 blockade in cancer. Nat Med 2021;27:1250–61.

62. Sharon S, Duhen T, Bambina S, et al. Explant Modeling of the Immune Environment of Head and Neck Cancer. Front Oncol 2021;11:611365.

63. Wu PC, Alexander HR, Huang J, et al. In vivo sensitivity of human melanoma to tumor necrosis factor (TNF)-alpha is determined by tumor production of the novel cytokine endothelial-monocyte activating polypeptide II (EMAPII). Cancer Res 1999;59: 205–12.

64. Mauldin IS, Wang E, Deacon DH, et al. TLR2/6 agonists and interferon-gamma induce human melanoma cells to produce CXCL10. Int J Cancer 2015; 137:1386–96.

65. Mauldin IS, Wages NA, Stowman AM, et al. Intratumoral interferon-gamma increases chemokine production but fails to increase T cell infiltration of human melanoma metastases. Cancer Immunol Immunother 2016;65:1189–99.

# Future Treatments in Melanoma

Kathryn Wells, DO[a], Vinesh Anandarajan, MD[a], James Nitzkorski, MD, FACS, FSSO[a],*

## KEYWORDS

- Melanoma • Immunotherapy • Intralesional therapy • Neoadjuvant therapy • Clinical trials

## KEY POINTS

- Melanoma management has evolved considerably over the past decade
- The head and neck surgeon caring for patients with melanoma should be aware of new and emerging therapies for melanoma.
- Neoadjuvant therapy is well understood in other cancers, and there is a promising role for its use in clinically detectable stage III melanoma.
- Intralesional therapy is an active area of research, with options including talimogene laherparepvec, tavokinogene telseplasmid, and PV-10.
- Combination therapy is an attractive option for further research in melanoma treatment.

## INTRODUCTION

Melanoma is a highly malignant tumor that arises from melanocytes, which are found in the basal layer of the epidermis. In the United States, the incidence of melanoma is 21.8 cases per 100,000 people, according to the Centers for Disease Control and Prevention.[1] Over the last decade, substantial therapeutic developments have revolutionized the treatment of malignant melanoma, especially among patients with advanced disease. Unprecedented sustained long-term survival is now possible among patients who were appropriate for hospice care just years ago.

Surgical extirpation of disease remains the mainstay of curative-intent treatment of malignant melanoma, and multimodality management of advanced and high-risk disease have dramatically improved. A more selective use of completion lymphadenectomy with routine ultrasonographic surveillance for sentinel-node positive patients has been shown to limit morbidity without compromising survival among patients with stage III melanoma.[2] In addition to surgical resection, immune checkpoint inhibitor therapy and targeted therapy have become commonplace among most multidisciplinary practices.

Other treatment modalities such as isolated limb perfusion and infusion, radiotherapy, interferon alfa, peginterferon alfa, and talimogene laherparepvec (TVEC) remain important tools in the war chest of therapeutic options. Despite dramatic improvements in the multimodality management of melanoma over the past decade, melanoma remains challenging to treat. Many patients with melanoma remain at risk for poor outcomes and death, and future developments in melanoma management remain critical and pertinent. Although a complete and thorough summary of all current investigations and trials for melanoma are beyond the scope of this text, this review should provide an overview of emerging therapeutics and concepts pertinent to the head and neck surgeon caring for patients with malignant melanoma.

[a] Department of Surgery, Vassar Brothers Medical Center, Nuvance Health, Dyson Center for Cancer Care, 45 Reade Place, 3rd Floor Surgical Oncology, Poughkeepsie, NY 12601, USA
* Corresponding author.
E-mail address: james.nitzkorski@nuvancehealth.org

Oral Maxillofacial Surg Clin N Am 34 (2022) 325–331
https://doi.org/10.1016/j.coms.2021.11.003
1042-3699/22/© 2021 Elsevier Inc. All rights reserved.

## GENE EXPRESSION PROFILING

Traditional clinicopathologic characteristics of a melanoma such as tumor thickness, ulceration, mitotic rate, and nodal status have historically been used to estimate risk of recurrence and guide recommendations for surgical treatment and adjuvant therapy. Although most patients are well served with these reliable tools, some patients with adequately resected nonmetastatic melanoma will in fact develop recurrent disease and some will indeed die from their disease. In recent years, adjuncts to traditional histopathologic testing have been developed. DecisionDx Melanoma (Castle Biosciences) is a gene expression profile test. This test uses real-time quantitative polymerase chain reaction to evaluate 28 prognostic and 3 control genes in order to create a tumor-specific signature of gene expression, rendering a more personalized assessment of risk. The test classifies patients into 4 categories of risk for developing metastatic disease. Its efficacy has been validated, identifying 80% of patients who had negative sentinel lymph node biopsy but went on to develop metastatic melanoma.[3] This gene expression profile test was shown to be an independent risk factor of metastasis among patients with melanoma.[4] Although the utilization of gene expression profiling to predict risk in melanoma is intriguing and promising, it remains investigational at the time of this writing.

## TREATMENT FOR HIGH-RISK RESECTED LOCAL DISEASE

Although most patients with nonmetastatic melanoma will survive their cancer, some patients with resected node-negative thick worrisome primary tumors are at risk for relapse. At least 11% of patients who present with stage II melanoma in the United States will experience relapse,[5] and melanoma-specific survival rate for patients with stage IIC melanoma is only 75% at 10 years.[6] As such, some patients with high-risk nonmetastatic melanoma may benefit from adjuvant therapy. Although adjuvant interferon-$\alpha$ has been shown to slightly improve outcomes among patients with high-risk (particularly ulcerated) melanoma,[7,8] toxicity concerns limit its use in the United States. There have been several contemporary trials designed for high-risk localized melanoma. One such trial is the Keynote 716 trial, which is currently enrolling. This 2-part phase III, randomized, double-blind study compares adjuvant pembrolizumab in patients with high-risk resected stage II melanoma with placebo. In part 1, patients are randomized to receive pembrolizumab or placebo.

In part 2, those who received placebo or those who completed the initial 17 cycles without recurrence after 6 months are eligible for 35 additional cycles.[9] Similarly, the Checkmate 76 trial is a phase III, double-blind, randomized controlled trial comparing adjuvant nivolumab with placebo in this high-risk population of patients with melanoma.[10] The NivoMela trial is also examining use of adjuvant nivolumab. Patients will be screened with genetic testing to determine those with increased risk of recurrence. Those with elevated risk will be randomized 2:1 into treatment versus observation. Those who are not high risk will be followed-up for 5 years in a third arm.[11] The primary endpoint for all 3 of these trials is recurrence-free survival, and results of these studies may change the management paradigm of high-risk localized melanoma after resection.

## NEOADJUVANT THERAPY

Neoadjuvant therapy has led to improved resectability and improved disease-free and overall survival rates in several types of cancer. Now that the benefit of targeted and immunotherapies for melanoma in both the advanced and adjuvant has been well established, it is only logical to investigate treatment of patients with resectable disease before surgery. Approximately 15% of patients with melanoma present with clinically evident stage III disease. These patients are at high risk for poor outcomes, and with clinically measurable disease these patients are ideal candidates for preoperative therapy. The OpACIN-neo trial published in 2018 was a phase II randomized controlled trial, which evaluated concurrent neoadjuvant ipilimumab and nivolumab in patients with stage III melanoma metastatic to lymph nodes. They demonstrated that 2 cycles of this combination therapy had a tolerable side-effect profile and produced a pathologic complete response in 77% of the group receiving this treatment regimen.[12] Although the small number of patients enrolled in this trial is limiting, this may provide a steppingstone for broader clinical applications of neoadjuvant immunotherapy.

The PRADO trial was a phase II extension cohort of the multicenter OpACIN-neo study, which evaluated response-driven subsequent therapy among patients with measurable clinically staged III disease. Each patient received a personalized approach to treatment depending on the presence of a pathologic complete response after neoadjuvant therapy. Ninety-nine patients with stage III melanoma received 2 cycles of ipilimumab and nivolumab, followed by resection of the index lymph node. If pathologic complete response was present with less than 10% viable tumor cells in the lymph node, therapeutic lymph node dissection and adjuvant therapy were omitted. Those with partial response underwent therapeutic lymph node dissection and were observed without adjuvant therapy. Patients with pathologic nonresponse, as defined by greater than 50% viable tumor cells in the specimen, underwent surgery followed by systemic adjuvant therapy. In total, 71% of patients experienced a response and 61% had a major response. Therapeutic lymph node dissection was omitted in 97% of patients with a major pathologic response. Immune-mediated adverse events occurred in 22% of patients during the treatment.[13] The PRADO trial suggests that among carefully selected patients, therapeutic lymph node dissection may be avoided if the response to preoperative therapy is robust. Long-term follow-up and larger trials will be necessary before any definitive conclusions can be made.

Preoperative therapy is also being applied to BRAF mutated melanoma. A phase II randomized controlled trial published in 2018 compared standard of care (surgery plus consideration for adjuvant therapy) with neoadjuvant and adjuvant therapy with dabrafenib and trametinib. This trial was a small study of 21 patients with resectable clinical stage III to IV melanoma. One-quarter of the patients demonstrated significantly longer event-free survival in the neoadjuvant group compared with the standard of care group.[14] Although this was a small trial with limited generalizability, it demonstrates feasibility in using targeted therapy in the preoperative setting.

Pembrolizumab is also being evaluated in the preoperative setting. A phase II randomized study (SWOG S1801) is currently recruiting to investigate the efficacy of pembrolizumab in high-risk (stage III/IV) melanoma. This trial will enroll 500 patients comparing adjuvant therapy alone with combination neoadjuvant/adjuvant therapy.[15]

In one small trial, a single dose of preoperative pembrolizumab was shown to produce a complete or near-complete response in almost 30% of patients treated before surgery.[16] Although promising, further research is necessary before neoadjuvant therapy can become mainstream. As of July 2021, 79 neoadjuvant clinical trials for melanoma were listed in ClinicalTrials.gov. To date, small patient populations and other challenges have limited the broad application of neoadjuvant therapy for melanoma at this time. In 2016, the International Neoadjuvant Melanoma Consortium (INMC) was established to help determine the best practices for conducting neoadjuvant trials in melanoma. The INMC has published comprehensive best practices recommendations for inclusion criteria, treatment duration, key endpoints, the role of genomic testing, and the collection and analysis of biospecimen.[17] Although neoadjuvant therapy for melanoma will almost certainly find a role, at this point treatment before resection remains investigational.

## ANTIANGIOGENIC THERAPY

Vascular endothelial growth factor (VEGF) is an important pathway for angiogenesis in tumor cells.[18] Bevacizumab, a VEGF inhibitor, has been investigated as a potential drug for patients with high-risk melanoma. The AVAST-M trial was conducted between 2007 and 2012 with 1343 patients randomized to receive adjuvant bevacizumab or observation. Patients had stage II or III melanoma and had already undergone resection. Although a minimal improvement in disease-free interval was seen, the treatment did not improve 5-year overall survival, which was 64% in both groups. Interestingly, a small trend toward improved survival was seen among BRAF mutant patients treated with bevacizumab.[19]

There is still interest in using VEGF inhibitors in combination with other agents as adjuvant therapy.[20] For example, one investigation combined ipilimumab with bevacizumab as therapy in patients with unresectable stage III or stage IV melanoma. Overall, there was an increase in efficacy in this specific phase I trial with combination therapy, so perhaps antiangiogenic treatment will find a place in the future.[20]

## INTRALESIONAL THERAPY

Intralesional therapy has long been of interest for unresectable cutaneous melanoma. As opposed to systemic treatment, intralesional therapy can be directly administered by a surgeon or medical oncologist in the clinic. This is distinctly advantageous given its relative ease, especially among patients who may need to travel some distance for specialized multidisciplinary care. In 1970, intratumoral Bacille Calmette-Guérin (BCG) injections were shown to induce an immune response. Substantial regression of injected cutaneous lesions, and even some abscopal regression of uninjected lesions, were seen among immunocompetent patients. Some of these patients remained free of disease for up to 6 years.[21] Significant toxicity limited BCG use, but what became clear in the 1970s was a clearly documented potential for immune-related and intralesional therapies to lead the path for subsequent discovery. One such currently approved therapy is intralesional

TVEC, an attenuated herpes simplex virus containing the granulocyte macrophage colony-stimulating factor (GM-CSF). The mechanism of this Food and Drug Administration–approved therapy is 2-fold—direct oncolysis by viral infection and lytic replication and also stimulation of immune response. Its efficacy is demonstrated in the OPTiM trial, a randomized phase III trial, with improved overall survival and durable response rate in the T-VEC group compared with intralesional GM-CSF alone.[22]

TVEC has also been evaluated in combination with other monoclonal therapies such as ipilimumab and pembrolizumab. A phase I study evaluating TVEC plus ipilimumab demonstrated 4 partial and 5 complete responses in a group of 19 patients, with an objective response rate of 50%,[23] and this led to a follow-up phase II trial of 198 patients with at least unresectable stage IIIB melanoma comparing TVEC plus ipilimumab and ipilimumab alone. The objective response rate in the combination group was 39% compared with 18% with ipilimumab alone, and the safety profile of combination therapy was similar to ipilimumab alone.[24] Pembrolizumab plus TVEC also had promising results in a phase I trial, demonstrating an objective response rate of greater than 50%,[25] but a larger follow-up phase II trial was recently terminated.[26] These treatment combinations are promising, but further studies are required with longer follow-up to determine if there are more durable response rates.

Another unique intralesional therapy is tavokinogene telseplasmid (TAVO). It relies on the well-characterized role of interleukin (IL)-12 in innate and adaptive immunity. IL-12 is a powerful proinflammatory cytokine, which has been investigated in several malignancies including melanoma. Systemic IL-12 administration causes severe toxicity, so systemic use is now mostly of historic interest. Intralesional IL-12 injection results in some objective response, but the response is brief and limited.[27] As opposed to intralesional and systemic administration of IL-12, TAVO is an intratumoral injection of plasmid IL-12 followed by electroporation, which results in increased and sustained elevation of IL-12 in the tumor microenvironment.[28] TAVO has been shown to regress both locally treated and distant (nontreated) lesions[28] with an abscopal effect. In a prospective phase II trial, 28 patients were treated with TAVO monotherapy. The objective overall response rate was 35.7% with a complete response rate of 17.9%. Response was identified not only in treated tumors but also in untreated distant tumors consistent with an immune-mediated abscopal effect. The treatment was relatively well tolerated,

with far less systemic toxicity when compared with traditional IL-12 therapy.[29] TAVO in combination with pembrolizumab has been shown to achieve a response in 41% of patients with advanced melanoma, with a 36% complete response rate among patients with low frequencies of checkpoint positive tumor infiltrating lymphocytes.[30] TAVO in combination with pembrolizumab is currently being studied in a larger phase II clinical trial.[31] Further studies with longer follow-up and larger study population will be required to demonstrate durable responses.

Lastly, intralesional Rose Bengal (PV-10) has been studied as an intralesional therapy. It is understood to work by transfusing directly across the cancer cell membrane and entering lysosomes leading to cell lysis. A phase I study demonstrated 48% objective response rate. A phase II study in 80 patients with unresectable stage III and stage IV melanoma who have failed multiple other therapies demonstrated a 51% overall response rate and a complete response rate of 26%. In addition, 8% of the patients in the study group had no evidence of disease at 52 weeks.[32] Intralesional therapies are a growing area of research in melanoma treatment. Used as monotherapy, or in combination with other treatments, surgeons involved in melanoma management should be familiar with intralesional therapies, as they could emerge as more important options for advanced melanoma.

## VACCINE FOR MELANOMA

In 1891, Dr William B. Coley, a surgeon in New York published a report in the Annals of Surgery describing 3 cases of malignant tumors regressing after the injection of streptococcal organisms.[33] For over a century, vaccination as a form of cancer treatment has continued to fascinate, while remaining largely insuperable. There have been multiple strategies used in melanoma vaccine development, including antigen-presenting cells, tumor antigens, or with direct modulation of the tumor itself.[34] To date, melanoma vaccines have unfortunately failed to demonstrate a positive impact on survival. However disappointing, vaccine research continues to hold potential. An open-label randomized phase II trial comparing mRNA vaccination with cemiplimab in anti-PD1-refractory/relapsed patients with advanced melanoma is currently underway. This trial will enroll 120 patients and is currently recruiting[35] in the United States and in Spain. In addition, early work using personal neoantigen vaccines for melanoma have been shown to induce persistent T-cell responses in melanoma, which may suggest on-target vaccine-induced tumor killing.[36] It is hoped that vaccination strategies in melanoma will add to our rapidly increasing portfolio of active agents for malignant melanoma.

## SUMMARY/DISCUSSION

In this section, we have describe a brief overview of current melanoma management. We have also discussed the paradigm shift toward increased use of targeted therapy and immune checkpoint inhibitor therapies and a more selective use of completion lymph node dissection. Over the past decade we have witnessed extraordinary and long overdue advances in melanoma medicine. These changes have been practice changing for surgeons, and most importantly they have been life changing for the patients we take care of. Nonetheless, some unfortunate patients with melanoma remain at risk for relapse and death. Further developments in gene expression profiling and identifying subsets of patients who may benefit from adjuvant therapy for stage II melanoma will only likely improve with time. Neoadjuvant therapy for melanoma is promising, but we have only begun to understand how it is best used. I suspect that intralesional therapy use will become more widespread and available with time. Melanoma vaccines have always been promising, but perhaps we are closer than ever to unlocking their potential. It is certainly an optimistic time to care for patients with melanoma, and I remain hopeful that even more optimism will be possible soon.

## CLINICS CARE POINTS

- Newer therapies have drastically improved survival for some patients with serious melanoma.

- Surgeons who take care of patients with melanoma should have an understanding of some of the emerging therapeutic agents available and should consider referral for clinical trials when appropriate.

- Although the mainstay of melanoma management has and will continue to be surgical, the importance of multidisciplinary management is more important now than ever before.

## DISCLOSURES

Dr J. Nitzkorski is a consultant for Oncosec.

## REFERENCES

1. Centers for Disease Control and Prevention. Melanoma Incidence and Mortality, United States–2012–2016. USCS Data Brief, no. 9. Atlanta, GA: Centers for Disease Control and Prevention, US Department of Health and Human Services; 2019.

2. Faries MB, Thompson JF, Cochran AJ, et al. Completion Dissection or Observation for Sentinel-Node Metastasis in Melanoma. N Engl J Med 2017;376(23):2211–22.

3. Gerami P, Cook RW, Russell MC, et al. Gene expression profiling for molecular staging of cutaneous melanoma in patients undergoing sentinel lymph node biopsy. J Am Acad Dermatol 2015;72(5):780–5.e3.

4. Gerami P, Cook RW, Wilkinson J, et al. Development of a Prognostic Genetic Signature to Predict the Metastatic Risk Associated with Cutaneous Melanoma. Clin Cancer Res 2015;21(1):175–83.

5. Research Emphasis | Division of Cancer Control and Population Sciences (DCCPS). Available at: https://cancercontrol.cancer.gov/research-emphasis. Accessed August 1, 2021.

6. Gershenwald JE, Scolyer RA, Hess KR, et al. Melanoma staging: Evidence-based changes in the American Joint Committee on Cancer eighth edition cancer staging manual. CA Cancer J Clin 2017;67(6):472–92.

7. Garbe C, Peris K, Hauschild A, et al. Diagnosis and treatment of melanoma. European consensus-based interdisciplinary guideline – Update 2016. Eur J Cancer 2016;63:201–17.

8. Eggermont A, Dummer R. The 2017 complete overhaul of adjuvant therapies for high-risk melanoma and its consequences for staging and management of melanoma patients - ClinicalKey. Eur J Cancer 2017;86:101–5.

9. Merck Sharp & Dohme Corp. Adjuvant Therapy With Pembrolizumab Versus Placebo in Resected High-Risk Stage II Melanoma: A Randomized, Double-Blind Phase 3 Study (KEYNOTE-716). clinicaltrials.gov. 2020. Available at: https://clinicaltrials.gov/ct2/show/NCT03553836. Accessed July 20, 2021.

10. Bristol-Myers Squibb. A Phase 3, Randomized, Double-Blind Study of Adjuvant Immunotherapy With Nivolumab Versus Placebo After Complete Resection of Stage IIB/C Melanoma. clinicaltrials.gov. 2021. Available at: https://clinicaltrials.gov/ct2/show/NCT04099251. Accessed July 20, 2021.

11. Schadendorf PD med D. Adjuvant Nivolumab Treatment in Stage II High-Risk Melanoma - A Randomized, Controlled, Phase III Trial With Biomarker-Based Risk Stratification. clinicaltrials.gov. 2021. Available at: https://clinicaltrials.gov/ct2/show/NCT04309409. Accessed July 21, 2021.

12. Rozeman EA, Menzies AM, van Akkooi ACJ, et al. Identification of the optimal combination dosing schedule of neoadjuvant ipilimumab plus nivolumab in macroscopic stage III melanoma (OpACIN-neo): a multicentre, phase 2, randomised, controlled trial. Lancet Oncol 2019;20(7):948–60.

13. First safety and efficacy results of PRADO: A phase II study of personalized response-driven surgery and adjuvant therapy after neoadjuvant ipilimumab (IPI) and nivolumab (NIVO) in resectable stage III melanoma. Available at: https://meetinglibrary.asco.org/record/185836/abstract. Accessed July 18, 2021.

14. Amaria RN, Prieto PA, Tetzlaff MT, et al. Neoadjuvant plus adjuvant dabrafenib and trametinib versus standard of care in patients with high-risk, surgically resectable melanoma: a single-centre, open-label, randomised, phase 2 trial. Lancet Oncol 2018; 19(2):181–93.

15. National Cancer Institute (NCI). A Phase II Randomized Study of Adjuvant Versus NeoAdjuvant Pembrolizumab (MK-3475) for Clinically Detectable Stage III-IV High-Risk Melanoma. clinicaltrials.gov. 2021. Available at: https://clinicaltrials.gov/ct2/show/NCT03698019. Accessed July 15, 2021.

16. Huang AC, Orlowski RJ, Xu X, et al. A Single Dose of Neoadjuvant PD-1 Blockade Predicts Clinical Outcomes in Resectable Melanoma. Nat Med 2019; 25(3):454–61.

17. Amaria RN, Menzies AM, Burton EM, et al. Neoadjuvant systemic therapy in melanoma: recommendations of the International Neoadjuvant Melanoma Consortium - ClinicalKey. Lancet Oncol 2019;20(7). Available at: https://www-clinicalkey-com.nuvanceremote.senylrc.org/#!/content/play Content/1-s2.0-S1470204519303328?returnurl=null&referrer=null. Accessed August 1, 2021.

18. Song Y, Fu Y, Xie Q, et al. Anti-angiogenic Agents in Combination With Immune Checkpoint Inhibitors: A Promising Strategy for Cancer Treatment. Front Immunol 2020;11. https://doi.org/10.3389/fimmu.2020.01956.

19. Corrie PG, Marshall A, Nathan PD, et al. Adjuvant bevacizumab for melanoma patients at high risk of recurrence: survival analysis of the AVAST-M trial. Ann Oncol 2018;29(8):1843–52.

20. Furukawa K, Nagano T, Tachihara M, et al. Interaction between Immunotherapy and Antiangiogenic Therapy for Cancer. Molecules 2020;25(17):3900.

21. Morton DL, Eilber FR, Holmes EC, et al. BCG Immunotherapy of Malignant Melanoma: Summary of a Seven-year Experience. Ann Surg 1974;180(4):635–41.

22. Andtbacka RHI, Collichio F, Harrington KJ, et al. Final analyses of OPTiM: a randomized phase III trial of talimogene laherparepvec versus granulocyte-macrophage colony-stimulating factor in unresectable stage III–IV melanoma. J Immunother Cancer 2019;7(1):145.

23. Puzanov I, Milhem MM, Minor D, et al. Talimogene Laherparepvec in Combination With Ipilimumab in Previously Untreated, Unresectable Stage IIIB-IV Melanoma. J Clin Oncol 2016;34(22):2619–26.

24. Chesney J, Puzanov I, Collichio F, et al. Randomized, Open-Label Phase II Study Evaluating the Efficacy and Safety of Talimogene Laherparepvec in Combination With Ipilimumab Versus Ipilimumab Alone in Patients With Advanced, Unresectable Melanoma. J Clin Oncol 2018;36(17):1658–67.

25. Ribas A, Dummer R, Puzanov I, et al. Oncolytic Virotherapy Promotes Intratumoral T Cell Infiltration and Improves Anti-PD-1 Immunotherapy. Cell 2017; 170(6):1109–19.e10.

26. Amgen A. Phase 1b/3, Multicenter, Trial of Talimogene Laherparepvec in Combination With Pembrolizumab (MK-3475) for Treatment of Unresectable Stage IIIB to IVM1c Melanoma (MASTERKEY-265/KEYNOTE-034). clinicaltrials.gov; . 2021. Available at: https://clinicaltrials.gov/ct2/show/NCT02263508. Accessed July 15, 2021.

27. Motzer RJ, Schwartz LH, Olencki T, et al. Phase I trial of subcutaneous recombinant human interleukin-12 in patients with advanced renal cell carcinoma. | Clin Cancer Res. 4(5). Available at: https://clincancerres.aacrjournals.org/content/4/5/1183.long. Accessed August 1, 2021.

28. Daud AI, DeConti RC, Andrews S, et al. Phase I Trial of Interleukin-12 Plasmid Electroporation in Patients With Metastatic Melanoma. J Clin Oncol 2008; 26(36):5896–903.

29. Algazi A, Bhatia S, Agarwala S, et al. Intratumoral delivery of tavokinogene telseplasmid yields systemic immune responses in metastatic melanoma patients. Ann Oncol 2020;31(4):532–40.

30. Algazi AP, Twitty CG, Tsai KK, et al. Phase II Trial of IL-12 Plasmid Transfection and PD-1 Blockade in Immunologically Quiescent Melanoma. Clin Cancer Res 2020;26(12):2827–37.

31. OncoSec Medical Incorporated. A Multicenter Phase 2, Open Label Study of Intratumoral Tavokinogene Telseplasmid (Tavo, PIL-12) Plus Electroporation in Combination With Intravenous Pembrolizumab in Patients With Stage III/IV Melanoma Who Are Progressing on Either Pembrolizumab or Nivolumab Treatment (Keynote 695) clinicaltrials.gov;. 2021. Available at: https://clinicaltrials.gov/ct2/show/NCT03132675. Accessed July 29, 2021.

32. Thompson JF, Agarwala SS, Smithers BM, et al. Phase 2 Study of Intralesional PV-10 in Refractory Metastatic Melanoma. Ann Surg Oncol 2015;22(7):2135–42.

33. Coley WB. Contribution to the Knowledge of Sarcoma. Ann Surg 1891;14(3):199–220.

34. Maurer D, Butterfield LH, Vujanovic L. Melanoma Vaccines: Clinical Status and Immune Endpoints. Melanoma Res 2019;29(2):109–18.

35. BioNTech SE. Open-Label, Randomized Phase II Trial With BNT111 and Cemiplimab in Combination or as Single Agents in Patients With Anti-PD1-Refractory/Relapsed, Unresectable Stage III or IV Melanoma. clinicaltrials.gov. 2021. Available at: https://clinicaltrials.gov/ct2/show/NCT04526899. Accessed July 29, 2021.

36. Hu Z, Leet DE, Allesøe RL, et al. Personal Neoantigen Vaccines Induce Persistent Memory T Cell Responses and Epitope Spreading in Patients with Melanoma. Nat Med 2021;27(3):515–25.

Printed and bound by CPI Group (UK) Ltd, Croydon, CR0 4YY

08/05/2025

01864713-0011